D0742368

BIRTH CONTROL

BIRTH CONTROL

Aharon W. Zorea

Health and Medical Issues Today

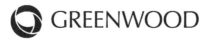

GREENWOOD

AN IMPRINT OF ABC-CLIO, LLC
Santa Barbara, California • Denver, Colorado • Oxford, England

Library of Congress Cataloging-in-Publication Data

Zorea, Aharon W.
  Birth control / Aharon W. Zorea.
    p. cm. — (Health and medical issues today)
  Includes bibliographical references and index.
    ISBN 978–0–313–36254–5 (hard copy : alk. paper) — ISBN 978–0–313–36255–2 (ebook)
  1. Birth control—United States. 2. Birth control—Government policy—United States. I. Title.
  HQ766.5.U5Z67   2012
  363.9'60973—dc23   2011043157

ISBN: 978–0–313–36254–5
EISBN: 978–0–313–36255–2

16 15 14 13 12   1 2 3 4 5

This book is also available on the World Wide Web as an eBook.
Visit www.abc-clio.com for details.

Greenwood
An Imprint of ABC-CLIO, LLC

ABC-CLIO, LLC
130 Cremona Drive, P.O. Box 1911
Santa Barbara, California 93116-1911

This book is printed on acid-free paper ∞

Manufactured in the United States of America

CONTENTS

SERIES FOREWORD

Every day, the public is bombarded with information on developments in medicine and health care. Whether it is on the latest techniques in treatment or research or on concerns over public health threats, this information directly affects the lives of people more than almost any other issue. Although there are many sources for understanding these topics—from websites and blogs to newspapers and magazines—students and ordinary citizens often need one resource that makes sense of the complex health and medical issues affecting their daily lives.

The *Health and Medical Issues Today* series provides just such a one-stop resource for obtaining a solid overview of the most controversial areas of health care in the twenty-first century. Each volume addresses one topic and provides a balanced summary of what is known. These volumes provide an excellent first step for students and laypeople interested in understanding how health care works in our society today.

Each volume is broken into several sections to provide readers and researchers with easy access to the information they need:

- Section I provides overview chapters on background information—including chapters on such areas as the historical, scientific, medical, social, and legal issues involved—that a citizen needs to intelligently understand the topic.
- Section II provides capsule examinations of the most heated contemporary issues and debates and analyzes in a balanced manner the viewpoints held by various advocates in the debates.
- Section III provides a selection of reference material, such as annotated primary source documents, a time line of important events,

and a directory of organizations that serve as the best next step in learning about the topic at hand.

The *Health and Medical Issues Today* series strives to provide readers with all the information needed to begin making sense of some of the most important debates going on in the world today. The series includes volumes on such topics as stem-cell research, obesity, gene therapy, alternative medicine, organ transplantation, mental health, and more.

INTRODUCTION

Artificial forms of birth control are now a common part of modern American life. As of 2010, the National Center for Health Statistics reported that 99 percent of sexually experienced women aged 15 to 44 have used some form of contraceptive at least once in their lives. Without the benefit of historical context, this simple statistic might suggest that birth control is now universally accepted and free from controversy. But a little more than a half century ago, when the first oral contraceptive was introduced, there were at least three states that outlawed the public sale and distribution of birth control. Just over a century ago, every church opposed birth control, every state had some prohibition against its dissemination as a form of obscenity, and certain sectors of the federal government actively monitored violations. The fact that birth control is now so common reflects a history of dramatic moral, social, political, and economic changes over the course of the twentieth century.

Even today, the predominance of birth control does not accurately reflect the level of controversy that is still associated with it. It is true that almost all women have used some form of birth control, but there are differences among methods and practice among sexually active women, suggesting greater diversity of opinion. At least 20 percent of sexually active women choose to permanently eliminate any chance of conception by sterilizing themselves or their partners. A majority of sexually active women (about 56 percent) remain open to conception in the future but choose one or more contraceptive methods. A large minority of sexually active women (about 20 percent) choose not to use any contraceptives at all. Although statistics provide little insight into personal motivation, the distribution of these results suggests a lack of consensus among

American men and women on the role of contraceptives in their lives. Despite the nearly universal experimentation, birth control remains controversial for a variety of moral, political, and economic reasons.

Historically, the practice and promotion of birth control has never been without some level of controversy. Contraceptives are not new, and references can be traced back to ancient times, with the earliest description of pessaries in Egypt dating from around 1850 BCE. Similar accounts found in ancient Roman, Indian and Chinese texts suggest that the practice was not limited to any single culture or era, but their scarcity also indicates that the dissemination of birth control information was usually limited or deliberately kept away from the mainstream of social discussion.

In more recent times, especially in the United States, birth control was regarded as immoral and unsafe. By modern standards, many methods used prior to the 1800s were unreliable and unsanitary. Such remedies included ritualistic charms, mercury-based potions, herbal mixtures, and pessaries made from any number of substances ranging from acacia gum to crocodile dung. Some of the social prohibitions against contraceptives certainly arose from twin concerns about consumer fraud and public safety. Doctors warned patients of the dangers of magical cures and their snake-oil salesmen, while the legal system prosecuted the purveyors of contraceptive manuals and devices under decency laws as an offense against the public order.

Yet even beyond the obvious risks to health and pocketbook, popular culture in the nineteenth century generally disapproved of artificial birth control as an offense against nature. The religious community viewed conception as a miracle that was only partially the result of human sexuality. The political community viewed population growth and its related increase in human labor as a key to national prosperity. For most Americans in the early 1800s, the idea of limiting family size seemed both selfish and a little unpatriotic. In this environment, birth control had very few advocates.

The turn of the twentieth century brought with it new perspectives on how scientific methods might be used to improve the social conditions of human society. Some social scientists argued that there was a correlation between poverty, criminality, and irresponsible reproduction. Others linked unregulated births to industrial exploitation and political oppression of both men and women. These were minority voices, but they were sufficient to shift the context of birth control away from questions of public decency toward new questions of public health.

By the mid-1920s, the question of legal dissemination of birth control information emerged as a matter of public debate. The majority of churches restated their traditional opposition, but they faced an increasing number of supporters from among the scientific community. Arguments in support of legal birth control varied—some relied on compassionate concern for mothers and others on the fear of unchecked immigrant populations, and still others feared the influence of organized religion on a free society. By the mid-1930s, the social environment had changed. More than half the protestant denominations came out in support of birth control on humanitarian grounds, and the remaining minority joined the Catholic Church in strong opposition. The scientific and legal community moved to open toleration.

The greatest pressures for public acceptance of contraceptives came during the 1950s as a result of an unusual confluence of technological breakthroughs and the emerging Cold War. Modern intrauterine devices and oral contraceptives transformed birth control into an almost sterile practice that involved little direct intrusion on sexual activity. At the same time, broad fears of unstable population explosions in the nonaligned world encouraged Western nations to pour millions of dollars into international family planning programs as part of their foreign policy objectives. By the late 1960s, birth control was legal and practiced by a vast majority of Americans of all faiths.

Although the 1960s ushered in a revolution in practice, it did not entirely resolve age-old questions of morality and ethics. The Catholic Church explicitly reaffirmed its opposition to contraception and abortion in 1968, and the 1973 Supreme Court decision of *Roe v. Wade* imbued the larger question of reproduction into political and social divisions. Since then, the trend in public support for birth control has not been entirely static one way or another. There was steady support for contraceptives as an alternative to abortion during the 1970s and 1980s, but the 1990s and 2000s saw a slight reversal in the trend as certain brands of birth control became increasing linked to abortion practice or ideology. The public continues to be mostly supportive, but the basis of support is no longer as consistent as it once was.

Since the 1970s, birth control has not only been legal in all 50 states, but it has also been partially subsidized by federal and state budgets. The addition of economic considerations opened the way for political controversy removed from obvious moral objections. Once in the political arena, the question of birth control became subject to partisan conflicts that remain a significant source of debate today. In 2011, strong political pressures led to proposals to completely defund Planned Parenthood and other agencies directly or indirectly linked to abortion services.

New advances in delivery methods in the 1990s also triggered a series of national debates highlighting the dynamic tension between the pharmaceutical industry, public demand, and the federal government's role in monitoring the safety and effectiveness of each new innovation. Consumer protection advocates raised questions about the amount of resources devoted to long-term testing and product liability. Certain developments, like long-acting contraceptives, raised questions about balancing the need for government policy designed to promote family planning against the individual's right to voluntarily halt their birth control method at will. Similarly, the introduction of multifunction contraceptive drugs led to national debates over how, where, and to whom birth control is marketed and sold.

Since the 1970s, birth control has also become a litmus test for various deeply rooted ideologies, including feminism, environmentalism, and the pro-family movements. Advocates and opponents may present contraceptive policy as a simple matter of public health, civil rights, or individual morality, but it is a difficult argument to make. The ideological diversity of American society prevents easy reconciliation between advocates and critics. Discussions over the direction of contraceptive technologies, over the manner in which they are marketed and sold, and over the degree of open access and the level of public subsidies all require a broad pluralist view that takes into account multiple perspectives. This book strives to provide a balanced discussion but leaves final conclusions to the personal reflection of the reader.

Historical Overview

CHAPTER 1

Types of Birth Control and Their Controversies

The intentional prevention and control of human conception is identified by many names but is today most commonly referred to as **birth control**. That particular term, however, dates back to 1914 when Margaret Sanger first used it in an essay she wrote for *Woman Rebel*. Prior to that point, advocates used much less explicit phrases that conveyed a sense of scientific objectivity, such as "reproductive control" or "birth regulation." Today, the term "birth control" is often used synonymously with "the pill," an oral contraceptive that synthesizes the progestin and estrogen hormones to chemically prevent conception. Chemical-based contraception, however, is only one form of birth control.

The specific distinctions between types of birth control are not trivial. As the president of Planned Parenthood, Alan Guttmacher, noted in the 1960s, much of the resistance to legalized and state-funded family planning policies arose from the stigma attached to **artificial birth control** devices. He claimed that all societies and all religions, from ancient to modern, have regulated human conception in some manner but that artificial birth control devices, especially the pill, seem more unnatural than other forms and thus face greater public scrutiny and resistance. Guttmacher argued that if the public recognized the commonalities between all forms of birth control, then the chemical versions would not seem so controversial.

Guttmacher focused on only a narrow point of dissension between opponents and advocates, but his larger point that semantic confusion underlay some of the conflict over birth control is well taken. Understanding the different methods of birth control will help to better clarify the premises and controversies of the many different voices in reproductive policy debates. Not all opponents of birth control policies oppose all contraceptives equally; some do not oppose contraceptives at all but oppose the manner in which they are promoted in society. Others support the premise of birth control as a civil right regardless of its specific mode. Still others oppose birth control only as a gateway to **abortion** and other policies that impact public morality.

NATURAL BIRTH CONTROL METHODS

Categorically, birth control can be divided between natural and artificial methods. Natural methods of contraception do not involve any outside chemical or device to implement and rely exclusively on the restraint of the individual sexual partners to abstain or limit sexual activity during times when conception is most likely. Artificial methods do not require individual restraint and instead rely on devices or chemicals to prevent pregnancy regardless of when the sexual activity occurs.

Since **natural birth control methods** require no technology, they have been practiced with varying degrees of popularity since the times of earliest civilization. Specific methods include restricting sexual intercourse to those days of postovulation infertility; extending breast-feeding to postpone ovulation (known as the **lactational amenorrhea method**); coitus interruptus, or early withdrawal before ejaculation; and nonvaginal intercourse. Of these methods, the first two have been endorsed by all religious groups. The latter two methods are referenced in the Old Testament— early withdrawal is indicated as the "sin of Onan," while nonvaginal intercourse is collectively labeled "sodomy"—and both practices were identified as sins. The fact that they are referenced at all nevertheless affirms Alan Guttmacher's assertion that some form of birth control was relatively common since ancient times.

Restricting sexual activity to those days of postovulation is often called **natural family planning** (NFP). It is the only method explicitly endorsed by the Catholic Church because it relies on individual restraint rather than artificial contraceptives. Typically, women ovulate a little more or less than two weeks after the last menstruation. The ovum is viable for only 12 to 24 hours, but sperm can survive for up to three days, so sexual intercourse in the days immediately prior to ovulation may still result in pregnancy. There are several NFP methods for determining when ovulation is complete and the ovum is no longer viable. One of the first techniques is called the "rhythm method" because women count the number of days since their last period to establish their body's rhythm of ovulation.

Couples need to refrain from intercourse during the days when the woman is most likely to be fertile. Since the length of each woman's ovulation cycle may be different, this method requires close tracking and may become unreliable if changes in the woman's health alter her ovulation rhythm.

More recent NFP techniques require daily monitoring of cervical mucus to establish ovulation cycles. In addition, special thermometers became available in the 1990s to measure basal body temperatures, which can also indicate days of ovulation. The **sympto-thermal method** combines these two techniques to achieve a very high probability of avoiding pregnancy. Technology provides greater precision in determining a woman's fertile days, but the NFP system still relies on couples to identify and refrain from sexual relations on the days that would most likely lead to pregnancy. For these reasons, some critics argue that the method is overly complicated, contrary to the needs of human passions, and generally unreliable. If the NFP methods are followed perfectly, the success rate is about the same or higher than artificial contraceptives. Critics argue, however, that the methods are rarely followed precisely. Moreover, other critics argue that couples should not have to restrain themselves to avoid pregnancy. It is that last point on which the moral issues surrounding birth control most focus.

Some religious groups, especially Catholics but also including more orthodox Jewish groups, distinguish between the types of natural birth control methods based on individual intent and the degree by which the action conforms to the natural order. For example, early withdrawal and nonvaginal intercourse are generally proscribed on the grounds that they involve unfaithful intent and are "unnatural"—despite the fact that the methods do not employ any additional devices or chemicals to prevent conception. The reasoning is based on a conviction that sexual intercourse is intended by God (and thus held by nature) as both a unitive act between a married couple and an act of procreation. Any attempt to sever the connection between unity and procreation involves a breach of faith in God's purpose for marriage and sexuality. In addition, interrupting the biological act of sexual intercourse requires deliberate human intent to avoid the natural consequences of union and is thus "unnatural." For its part, nonvaginal intercourse is unnatural because it misuses parts of the body for purposes that would not occur in nature without deliberate human intention.

These moral distinctions between natural birth control methods depend heavily on specific religious presumptions. Not only do they presume God's personal involvement in defining the laws of nature, but they also assume that God holds man accountable for abiding by them. The

Catholic position, for example, begins with an assumption that all human actions, including sexuality, are governed by revealed and natural laws, which humans must respect. Not all religious traditions agree on natural law or the intent of human reproduction, and these differences account for the spectrum of positions within the religious community over the appropriateness of natural or artificial birth control methods, including related issues of extramarital relations, **sterilization**, and abortion. For nonreligious groups, these objections find less meaning since they do not recognize any such presuppositions of sexuality. Even among advocates of birth control, differing religious preconceptions often account for a wide spectrum of viewpoints.

The moral debate over birth control involves more than pragmatic discussions of resource allocation, access, or health concerns. The conflicting positions involve deeply embedded issues of teleology and human nature and are rarely resolved through compromise. These philosophical differences likely underlay most of the other controversies related to birth control policies, but policymakers require more quantifiable justifications to support their positions. These moral differences tend to manifest themselves in practical debates over specific technologies, which invariably include questions of resource allocation, access, and health concerns.

EARLY ARTIFICIAL BIRTH CONTROL METHODS

Artificial birth control methods require some technological assistance, whether in the form of a pill, an ointment, or a device. Any technology used to prevent conception, regardless of its form, is called a **contraceptive**. The sophistication of the method depends on the current level of technology, but references to spermicidal ointments and uteral barriers (known as **pessaries**) can be dated back to classical times. These ancient folk remedies often involved combinations of natural acids, such as those found in fruits, saps, or other plant extracts. Although occasionally successful in killing or blocking some of the sperm during intercourse, their effectiveness was unpredictable, and the side effects could be painful, including rashes, inflammation, and other infections. Experiments with oral contraceptives during the Middle Ages, often described as potions, utilized arsenic or mercury, resulting in much more dangerous reactions. These methods, however, were not based on scientific experimentation and frequently required special incantations for the promised effect.

The **condom** might be considered the first science-based contraceptive, but it arose in the early sixteenth century in Paris initially as a protection against sexually transmitted diseases. Some references to the use of

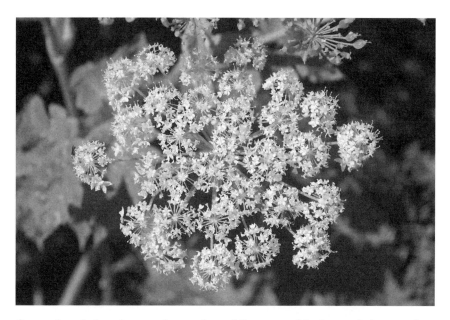

Queen Anne's lace is one of a number of flowers and herbs used since ancient times in concoctions intended to prevent pregnancy. (© Weldon Schloneger | Dreamstime.com)

animal membranes date back to ancient Egypt, but in the modern era, condoms were first constructed out of fine cloth. The use of condoms for contraceptive purposes did not become common until the mid-seventeenth century, nearly 200 years later.

Scientists did not directly tackle contraceptive technology until they were inspired to do so by the English economist Thomas Malthus. Although personally opposed to the use of artificial birth control, Malthus nevertheless warned of a pending catastrophe when the demands of increasing population outstripped the agricultural capabilities for sustaining it. His more radical disciples used the threat of overpopulation to push for broad education programs that taught women how to avoid pregnancy. In 1823, neo-Malthusian reformer and trade unionist Francis Place handed out flyers describing how to use sea sponges as an inexpensive pessary. Other similar reformers advocated vaginal douches, combined with a variety of spermicidal solutions to build the basis for what would later become a more science-driven contraceptive industry in Europe and the United States.

In 1843, Charles Goodyear invented the process called vulcanization, which made rubber more flexible and elastic. This technology gradually found its way into contraceptives and over the course of the next century eventually led to the invention of cervical caps, **diaphragms**, and later to rubber condoms. As technology improved, the expense of specific devices declined, and public access to more effective methods of artificial birth control increased proportionally.

Aside from the moral issues that can arise with all artificial birth control methods, the primary points of dissension rising from the specific use of condoms or uteral barrier devices deal with questions of male responsibility and ease of access for women. Some feminists and moralists contend that greater access to condoms encourages more irresponsibility among men. Condoms are marketed as both a protection against sexually transmitted diseases and as a birth control method, but they are imperfect and can sometimes fail in both objectives. Undo focus on condoms as a single solution against both disease and pregnancy might encourage patterns of risky behaviors. By contrast, uteral barriers only act as contraceptives and offer no protection against diseases. Some critics contend that they are cumbersome to use and they place too much responsibility for birth control on the woman alone.

INTRAUTERINE DEVICES

The next major innovation for female contraceptive devices came in 1909, when German physician Richard Richter invented the first **intrauterine device** (IUD), which was a ring-shaped device made of silkworm gut. When inserted into the uterus through the cervix, the IUD prevented conception. The idea apparently came from an ancient practice among Bedouin traders who inserted pebbles into the uterus of their camels to prevent pregnancy during long caravans. Richter's invention was later modified and marketed in 1928 by another German scientist, Ernst Grafenberg, who wrapped silk threads around a more stable silver ring.

Neither Richter nor Grafenberg knew exactly how the IUD worked, but the results were more successful than previous devices, such as sponges or douches. Grafenberg believed that the IUD irritated the uterus, causing inflammation and making conditions lethal for the sperm. He later added copper to trigger greater reactions, resulting in higher rates of contraception. These reactions, however, also resulted in other complications, such as infections, pelvic inflammatory disease, ectopic pregnancy, and long-term (or permanent) infertility.

Researchers later conjectured that irritation of the uterus was not essential for the IUD to be successful. In the late 1950s, several private doctors in New York City introduced a number of plastic versions of Grafenberg's

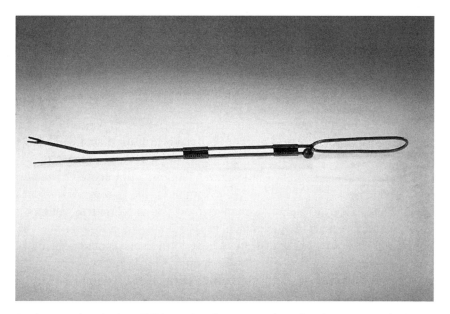

An intrauterine device (IUD) works after conception, denying a newly fertilized embryo the ability to implant and grow in the lining of the uterus. The Dalkon Shield was introduced on the American market in 1971 by A. H. Robins Company. It was a faulty IUD that became the subject of a law case and created widespread speculation about the effectiveness and safety of IUDs. The litigation case arose from allegations that the Dalkon Shield caused pelvic inflammatory disease, frequently resulting in infertility. More than 3.6 million devices were sold in the United States before it was removed from the market in 1974. Over 400,000 claims were made against A. H. Robins, and nearly $3 billion was eventually paid out in damages. (Photo by SSPL/Getty Images)

ring, each emphasizing the shape rather than the material alone as the active component. Lazar Marguilies introduced a spiral or coil-shaped IUD in 1958. In 1968, Howard Tatum introduced a large T-shaped IUD, but its size created complications, such as intestinal pain and bleeding. Later that same year, a Chilean doctor, Jaime Zipper, combined a little copper with the new T shape to create a smaller device with greater contraceptive effectiveness.

The IUD industry suffered a major blow after the A. H. Robins Company marketed the **Dalkon Shield** in 1971. It was pulled from the market three years later after more than 100 women experienced spontaneous abortions and seven women died from complications. The Food and Drug Administration (FDA) suspended specific support for the Dalkon Shield but did not prohibit the IUD as a birth control method.

A second-generation, copper and plastic–based IUD was developed in 1976 and still maintains a large market worldwide.

In the 1970s, Chinese scientists developed a stainless-steel ring that was intended to be less likely to lead to secondary infections. About 100 million women were required to use the steel IUD ring as part of China's strict population control policies. But by the 1990s, the country banned the steel IUD because there was still a 10 percent conception rate, indicating that the choice of material did have an impact on the device's effectiveness.

Today, IUDs have a very high success rate as a contraceptive method and are deemed safe by the FDA. Nevertheless, the two primary issues specifically related to IUD use involve questions of women's health and questions of voluntary use. Since scientists are still not absolutely certain how the IUD works, the question of long-term hazards cannot be fully closed. Although the Dalkon Shield does not represent modern IUDs, it nevertheless contributed to misconceptions and suspicions among the general public about IUD safety. In addition, IUDs can function for up to five years, with contraceptive effects sometimes lasting long after the devices have been removed. In the 1970s, cases were reported where IUDs were inserted into minority clients of public health clinics without their knowledge or without their fully informed consent. Some feminists and minority activists who might otherwise support artificial contraception devices were strongly opposed to the heavy-handed use of IUDs as a social welfare policy.

HORMONAL-BASED CONTRACEPTIVES

Perhaps the most significant innovation in contraceptive technology came with the invention of a scientifically tested oral contraceptive that combined progestin and estrogen hormones to prevent ovulation. The drug ensures that the ovum is never released to the ovaries so that pregnancy cannot occur. This hormone synthesis came in the form of a pill that women would have to take every day. After 21 days, the woman would stop taking the hormones to allow for the menstruation process. Since the method required regularity, some women took a placebo pill during the seven days prior to menstruation to maintain the habit of daily dosing. Compared to the variety of barrier methods that dominated the market until the 1960s, this science-based oral contraceptive seemed remarkably trouble free. It quickly became known simply as **the pill**.

The FDA approved the progestin/estrogen combination in 1960, but it had been under development for more than a dozen years prior. Shortly after World War II, several family planning organizations began working on an "anovulent" pill—one that would prevent ovulation. Research was undertaken by at least two labs working in tandem. Clarence Gamble headed the Committee on Maternal Health, while the Committee on Human Reproduction funded research by Gregory Pincus, John Rock, and Christopher Tietze. By the mid-1950s, the drug was ready for testing. Since several states still outlawed the sale of birth control products, the hormone combination was initially submitted for regulatory approval in 1957 as a therapy for menstrual disorders and infertility. It did not receive approval as a contraceptive until 1960.

Within a dozen more years, another innovation in oral contraceptives was introduced with the **minipill** in 1973. This progestin-only hormone acted as a chemical-based barrier method that reduces and thickens the cervical mucus to prevent sperm from reaching the uterus. It does not prevent ovulation, but it bypasses the need to insert any physical device into the cervix. It also creates a toxic environment, preventing the ovum from attaching to the uterus wall. The failure rate is slightly more than with the combined pill, but the side effects were less pronounced.

The period between 1960 and 1973 first transformed and then hardened popular positions on birth control. From a practical standpoint, the simple convenience and routine of taking a single oral contraceptive pill stood in stark contrast to the intrusive requirements of previous methods. For a society that did not like to speak of sexuality, the instructions for inserting a sponge, diaphragm, or cervical cap or for fitting a condom heightened the potential obscenity of birth control. While the IUD eliminated the requirement that the contraceptive be set in place before each and every sexual act, it still required a visit to a clinic to ensure proper insertion and periodic return visits to ensure that it remained in place. These inconveniences, while relatively minor, magnified the "unnatural" aspects of artificial birth control methods and played some role in explaining the resistance some women had to learning about or using birth control.

The pill form was itself a symbol of technological progress in medical science. Some of the prior reservations that women may have had with the obscenity of birth control were sidestepped by the sanitary simplicity of a single pill. The oral contraceptive no longer required deliberate preparation for a specific act of sexual intercourse. In addition, the daily dosage helped further associate birth control as an ordinary medical supplement and not as sex-related device. The General Board of the National Council of Churches of Christ proclaimed in a statement in 1961 that "couples are free to use the gifts of science for conscientious family limitation." Other advocates of birth control promoted the pill as a scientific breakthrough for women's health, and opponents had a difficult time countering the axiomatic attraction of medical progress.

Critics of the new oral contractive were slower to coalesce than the supporters. After the initial introduction in 1960, some observers believed that the Catholic Church would follow the lead set by many Protestant denominations by supporting birth control as a means of limiting family size and controlling poverty. They were surprised, though, when Pope Paul VI issued an encyclical in 1968, titled *Humanae Vitae*, that explicitly forbade the use of artificial contraceptives. Initial reaction among Catholics was mixed, including some splinter groups who explicitly rejected it and a much larger number who quietly ignored it. Nevertheless, the official teaching was explicit, and many Catholic leaders launched a renewed attack on the prevalence of artificial birth control as an example of moral decline in our modern culture.

The opposition to oral contraceptives became more steadfast in 1973 after the introduction of the progestin-only minipill. Unlike the **combination pill**, some critics feared that the minipill was a potential **abortifacient**, which induced an embryonic abortion if sperm managed to successfully pass into the uterus and fertilize the ovum and was later unable to attach itself to the uterus. Since Catholics teach that life begins at conception, then users of the minipill could potentially be destroying life without knowing or intending to do so. The question of what the minipill actually does remains very difficult to answer. As recently as 2006, researchers were unable to conclusively rule out whether progestin-only hormones prevented implantation of the ovum or prevented conception. Religious-based sensitivity to potential abortifacients remains a major issue for some critics of birth control. For many Catholics, the pill symbolized a gateway to abortion in much the same way that it also symbolized technological innovation for its supporters.

LONG-ACTING HORMONE-BASED CONTRACEPTIVES

Beginning in the 1990s, the contraceptive industry expanded in a variety of new technologies. One of the most significant, from a marketing perspective, was also one of the most controversial. In 1990, the FDA approved the **Norplant System** as a long-term contraceptive device. It was **hormonal based**, but it did not require daily dosing. Instead, the device consisted of six plastic rods filled with a new contraceptive steroid called **levonorgestrel**, which is a synthetic form of progestin. When inserted into a woman's upper arm, the rods released very low doses of the hormone for up to five years. Women no longer needed to take daily pills, nor did they need to undergo the more intrusive procedure for inserting an IUD.

At the time it was introduced, the Norplant System was hailed as a reversible alternative to sterilization. There were, however, some noticeable shortcomings. The rods required only a 10-minute procedure for insertion, but extraction was much more difficult and sometimes left scarring. As a progestin-based hormone, the expected side effects were very similar to the minipill. The primary difference was that women could suspend use of the minipill if the side effects became more than they were comfortable with. The Norplant was relatively difficult to extract, and it released its hormones continually. Many women complained of more pronounced reactions, including headaches, migraines, tenderness in the breasts, weight gain, nausea, anxiety, unwanted hair growth, and acne. Most significant, some women suffered from enlarged ovaries and ovarian cysts.

Production of the Norplant System was discontinued in 2002, but its introduction highlighted some controversial issues related to any **long-acting hormone-based contraceptives**. The first issue had to do with women's health. When the combination pill was introduced in 1960, most advocates, including Alan Guttmacher, "emphatically" denied any risks of cancer from the new drug. Nevertheless, by the 1970s, other researchers recognized the possible correlation between oral contraceptive use and increased risks of cancer. These risks were more pronounced among women who smoked and among women with family histories of breast cancer. Later research also indicated that women who started using oral contraceptives in their teens experienced higher risks of breast cancer, though those risks leveled off after 10 years of not taking the pill. Some activists argued that market pressures to introduce more convenient oral contraceptives forced women to take unnecessary risks to their health because drugs were introduced to the market without sufficient study into possible side effects. These critics became more vocal in the late 1990s, when women began experiencing more pronounced side effects while using the longer-acting hormone-based contraceptives.

The second issue that the Norplant System helped direct national attention to was the question of **voluntariness**. A woman who takes an oral contraceptive in a daily dose is able to decide every morning if she wants to continue her birth control method or discontinue it. An implant that is difficult to extract requires women to wait until her scheduled surgical appointment. Meanwhile, the patient would have to endure any uncomfortable side effects while she waited. To a lesser extent, these problems were also present for women who chose to use IUDs, but the prevalence of endocrine-related disorders caused the long-acting hormone-based contraceptives to receive more negative attention.

Within years of Norplant, other long-acting hormone-based contraceptives were introduced, including an injectable version of the minipill called **Depo-Provera**, which used a synthetic progesterone hormone called medroxyprogesterone. Its primary advantage was that it could be easily administered at a clinic with no embarrassing procedures and would last three months. The side effects were less noticeable than the Norplant System, affected fewer users, and required no extraction. All the disadvantages were related to questions of public health care policies, particularly with regard to how contraceptives were administered in public health clinics serving lower-income communities.

Since the 1950s, family planning organizations were closely linked to population control agendas. In the 1960s, many public welfare policies included family planning components, such as education and subsidized contraceptives, as a weapon in the war on poverty. This association with birth control and government control of certain population triggered some vocal reactions in the late 1970s, especially among African American and Hispanic civil rights leaders who alleged that the government was using family planning policies to kill off their communities. These reactions were especially focused on state-funded sterilization policies, which appeared to target minority women more than white or middle- or high-income women.

By the 1990s, the debate over voluntary use of birth control became politicized when allegations surfaced that some welfare recipients entering community health clinics for routine checkups might receive a contraceptive injection without being fully informed. Unlike the pill, which required self-administering, or the IUD, which required intrusive insertion, an injectable contraceptive might be administered without the patient knowing of its actual purpose. The instances of abuse were mostly hypothetical, but the potential for civil rights conflicts led to significant policy debates over how access to birth control should and should not be mandated. Significantly, these conflicts were not pitted between moral opponents of contraceptives but were most pronounced among those who were otherwise the strongest supporters of artificial birth control methods.

"EMERGENCY" CONTRACEPTIVES

In 1980, the French biochemist Etienne-Emile Baulieu developed a steroid that blocked the effects of progesterone, which is a necessary hormone for the development of embryos in the uterus. This antihormone was code named RU 486 and later marketed as **Mifepristone**. The French government approved of the drug as a nonsurgical abortion alternative in 1988. President Bill Clinton pushed for lifting the ban on its importation in 1992, and the FDA granted conditional approval in 1996. It is usually sold in a pill form but can also be injected by a clinician or taken as a liquid (known as methotrexate).

Mifepristone is not a contraceptive. It is an abortifacient, which works after the ovum has been fertilized. Abortion providers often refer to non-surgical abortions as "chemical abortions" or "medical abortions." Abortion opponents were strongly opposed to the legalization of mifepri-stone and its generic versions because they believed that the pill form could be self-administered with little or no oversight and may encourage women to use abortions as they might use contraceptives without recognizing the significant moral differences between preventing and ending pregnancy. Some groups that strongly support access to birth control are equally strongly opposed to abortifacients. Their support for artificial contraception is often based on the promise that birth control will negate any need or demand for abortion. Supporters of mifepristone argued that nonsurgical abortions are safer than surgical abortions and could more reliably end pregnancy at very early stages of development before a surgical abortion becomes necessary.

In 1999, the FDA approved a contraceptive that was difficult to distinguish from an abortifacient. This pill, containing high levels of levonorgestrel, was marketed under the name of **Preven (Plan B)** and was described as an **"emergency contraceptive"** because women could take the drug immediately after sexual intercourse and still reduce the risk of pregnancy by up to 80 percent. Within seven years and after three separate applications, Plan B was approved by the FDA for over-the-counter sales without a prescription.

Critics argued that Plan B was not a contraceptive but rather an abortifacient, which prevented implantation of the fertilized ovum. Researchers have been unable to deny or affirm the charge, but most evidence indicates that the postcoital contraceptive works by killing or blocking the sperm before it gains access to the ovum. Contraception is most likely if the pill is taken prior to the day of ovulation because the progestin hormone can suppress the mid-cycle leuteinizing hormone surge that triggers ovulation. In addition, it can thicken the cervix mucus within nine hours and alkalinize the uterine cavity fluid within five hours. The effect is to block access of the sperm yet to reach the cervix and then kill any sperm that had previously arrived. Nevertheless, if sexual intercourse occurs on the day near or before ovulation, the levonorgestrel hormone does not appear to stop fertilization, and as a result, women can still become pregnant after use about 20 percent of the time.

There is as yet no conclusive way to assess if the hormone prevents implantation, so it is impossible to determine if these postcoital contraceptives are also abortifacients. Despite the lack of quantifiable evidence on the subject, postcoital, or "emergency," contraceptives remain very controversial because of their association with mifepristone and abortion. The moral debates extend beyond those who oppose artificial birth control on principle but also include those who otherwise support contraceptives but strongly oppose abortion.

HOW DID BIRTH CONTROL GET ON TELEVISION?

The first legal condom commercial aired in San Francisco in January 1987. It followed the rise of public concern over the spread of HIV/AIDS cases in the United States, so the ad emphasized disease prevention more than birth control. The first oral contraceptive ad was aired in Texas two years later but in a limited market. For several years, only a few local stations aired commercials for over-the-counter contraceptives, such as condoms or contraceptive sponges.

Broadcasters resisted contraceptive commercials for several reasons, but few of those reasons were explicitly written into law. In part, local stations feared public protests against violations of expected standards of decency. In part also, broadcasters feared legal penalties levied by the Federal Communications Commission (FCC). The problem was that there were no clear boundaries defining the decency of birth control. Based on the Federal Communications Act of 1934, the FCC has authority to regulate all public airwaves, and it prohibits obscene material and indecent speech. The FCC developed general guidelines to define obscenity, but birth control did not easily fit into the calculus. The National Association of Broadcasters voluntarily banned contraceptive advertising during the 1970s, but individual broadcast stations had some freedom to deviate if they chose to.

The FCC is selective in its enforcement, and public reaction was often more determinative than the general guidelines. In an effort to avoid censorship, the FCC does not prohibit specific content from being shown; it can penalize stations for airing obscene or indecent material only after the fact, meaning that the FCC regulations require proactive enforcement for the standards to be meaningful. In addition, the FCC has jurisdiction over only content transmitted over the public airwaves and regulates only content aired between the hours of 6:00 A.M. and 10:00 P.M. The increasingly popular cable, satellite, and Internet providers are exempt from FCC oversight.

In addition to the decency standards of the FCC, contraceptive manufacturers faced disclosure requirements set forth by the Food and Drug

Administration (FDA). Prior to 1990s, prescription drugs were rarely advertised on television because the required disclosure of all potential harmful side effects often made the drug less marketable. But in 1989, Pharmacia & Upjohn broke into the television market with a pioneering ad campaign for its prescription-based hair restoration drug Rogaine. For two years, Rogaine commercials sidestepped FDA requirements by never indicating what the drug was for. Instead, the ads showed scene after scene of satisfied people thanking Rogaine but never explaining why. The commercial ended with a toll-free number to call for more information. The strategy worked, and Rogaine became one of the fastest-growing products among prescription drugs. Within two years, Pharmacia & Upjohn was able to shift strategies and explicitly identify Rogaine, including the full disclosure information. By that time, however, Rogaine's name recognition was so strong that the accompanying warnings had little impact on the marketing effectiveness.

Pharmacia & Upjohn launched another national television campaign in 1997 for its injectable contraceptive Depo-Provera. The company avoided the twin dangers of full disclosure (for the FDA) and the appearance of obscenity (for the FCC) by filling its commercial with images of babies and families and no sexual innuendo. Birth control was discussed specifically but scientifically, and the disclosure information actually helped the ads avoid any appearance of indecency. The strategy was successful and was quickly imitated by other contraceptive manufacturers. By 2009, contraceptive commercials were aired on almost any channel, during any time of day, with few limits on explicit references to sexual activity.

RECENT INNOVATIONS AND MARKETING

The marketing of artificial contraceptives changed dramatically in the late 1990s. The increase in public access to cable and satellite providers and the rapid growth of access to the Internet combined to change the way in which the Federal Communications Commission chose to enforce its decency standards. Contraceptive manufactures took advantage of the moment to market their products directly to the public rather than through doctors' referrals. New advertising strategies increased public demand, and in turn, the industry responded with innovative contraceptive products customized for specific market segments.

The increase in public marketing naturally increased the demand for new contraceptive innovations. By 2000, the number of contraceptive products increased significantly. An injectable version of the combination pill was marketed under the name **Lunelle**, which mixed synthesized forms of progestin and estrogen. The injection lasted only a month, and women had to make monthly appointments at a clinic to receive them. A year later, the **Ortho Evra** patch was developed that released low doses of the combination hormone synthesis into the bloodstream for a week at a time. They could be self-administered and applied to the lower abdomen or upper body. More important, the patch could be removed by the woman at any time with no clinical assistance. In the same year, the IUD was updated when **NuvaRing** was introduced. It combined the physical characteristics of Grafenberg's ring with the chemical effects of the combination pill. The flexible plastic ring was inserted below the cervix and released low doses of progestin and estrogen for three weeks, to be removed just prior to menstruation.

In addition to extended durations of effectiveness, pharmaceutical companies also introduced multipurpose contraceptives that address problems not related to birth control. In 2003, the FDA approved **Seasonale**, which is a low-dose daily combination pill that reduces the rate of menstruation to once every three months. The need for birth control was presumed, and the main emphasis of the ad campaign was the contraceptives' ability to minimize monthly periods. In 2007, Wyeth Pharmaceuticals introduced **Lybrel**, which eliminated the need for menstruation altogether, with a low-dose combination pill that can be taken 365 days with no placebo pills.

Earlier in 2003, the FDA also approved the use of a synthetic progestin called **Drospirenone**, which could also be used as a treatment for acne and symptoms of **premenstrual dysphoric disorder**, including backaches, bloating, irritability, and mood swings. It was marketed by Berlex Laboratories under two names, a 28-day cycle called **Yasmin**, and a 24-day cycle called **Yaz**. They were featured in television commercials with young girls excitedly explaining what "a difference a little chemistry can make." The ads downplayed references to birth control and emphasized relief from pimples, cramps, bloating, and weight gain. Later that year, the FDA ordered the manufacturer to stop running the ads because they failed to remind viewers of the risks of blood clots, heart attacks, strokes, and other symptoms related to increased potassium levels. In 2009, a class-action suit was filed claiming the drug manufacturer put women at risk of serious injury because they exaggerated benefits and failed to adequately warn them of the potential side effects. Despite the criticism, Yasmin and Yaz were the best-selling oral contraceptive pills in the United States, controlling 29 percent of the market in 2008.

The influx of new birth control alternatives helped to greatly expand the size and power of the contraceptive industry. Their presence on television, however, also resurrected old criticisms as well as some new controversies relating to marketing strategies. Morality-driven critics argue that the new contraceptive ads target younger markets, including age-groups that should not be sexually active. Multipurpose contraceptives use less controversial problems, such as monthly menstruation and teen acne, to redirect public attention away from the moral and emotional dangers that accompanies risky lifestyles of uncommitted or casual sexual activity. Some woman advocacy groups also voiced concerns that aggressive marketing campaigns minimized consumer awareness of potentially harmful health risks of long-term usage. These critics feared that overly quick FDA approvals used women as test subjects for a pharmaceutical industry that is concerned mostly about expanding its market share.

By contrast, contraceptive manufacturers and their supporters responded that the drugs are safe and that consistent use of birth control helps safeguard the physical and emotional well-being of modern women and families. They contend that opponents base their criticisms on archaic standards of morality, which do not reflect modern consensus, and they may actually be harmful for the independent development of young people. Other women advocacy groups argue strongly that the right to free and easy access to all reproductive choices (from birth control to abortion) should be safeguarded, and therefore increased advertising of birth control actually helps promote women's awareness of their options.

The increase in televised marketing of contraceptives triggered a minor battle in the larger cultural war over public morality, and it may contribute to future policy debates over new definitions of obscenity. But unlike the situation of the 1950s and 1960s, the advocates of birth control hold a deferential position in the debate. It is up to the critics to generate the public opposition necessary to change current practices.

STERILIZATION

The last form of birth control, sterilization, belongs in a category that is separate from natural and artificial contraceptive methods. Whether through surgery or chemical reaction, sterilization permanently eliminates the possibility of fertility and thus does not "control" birth. The sterilization procedure for men is called a **vasectomy** because the vas deferens ducts that carry the sperm from the testes are cut and fused or tied together. For women, the procedure is called **tubal ligation** because it blocks the fallopian tubes, which carry the ovum from the ovaries to the uterus. There are two methods of tubal ligation: **minilaparotomy** and laparoscopy. The first requires a doctor to make an incision in the abdomen and then draw out the fallopian tubes to be tied together. The second, more recent method requires much smaller instruments with video technology that allow doctors to fuse the fallopian tubes with an electric current (or a band/clip) without opening the abdominal cavity.

The **Essure System** is a third option for female sterilization approved by the FDA in 2002, and it does not require extensive surgery. Doctors use a catheter to implant a small metal implant in the fallopian tubes that creates scar tissue that blocks the ovum as effectively as if they were cut. Women must wait three months for the tissue to form and until placement is confirmed by an X-ray. Women should expect that the final results of both surgical and nonsurgical tubal ligations are permanent. Although microsurgical technique may reverse both vasectomy and tubal ligation procedures, the rates of success are so low that men and women must treat them as irreversible.

Despite its permanence, sterilization is not perfectly effective for preventing conception. Both male and female procedures have a small failure rate of about 1 in 100—about half that expected through artificial and natural contraceptive methods when perfectly implemented. In some cases, the failures may be due to surgical error, equipment malfunction, or a natural healing process. Some men discovered they had reestablished connection between the vas deferens, and some women experienced recanalization of the fallopian tubes between the ovaries and uterus. Both reactions require a second surgery if the patients want to remain sterilized.

The only guaranteed method of sterilization is castration, or the complete removal of the male testicles or the female ovaries. Castration is not viewed as a birth control method for men because it may (though not always) lead to a diminished ability to achieve an erection. For women, removal of the ovaries (known as a **bilateral salpingo-oophorectomy**) has no effect on a woman's ability to engage in sexual activity, but it is a serious surgery. It triggers immediate surgical menopause and is usually performed only in conjunction with a hysterectomy as a treatment for various hormone-sensitive cancers.

The side effects of sterilization can be problematic. Unlike **castration**, sterilization does not end the production of hormones in the reproductive system. Women continue their cycles, often with heavier menstrual bleeding as a result of elevated levels of estrogen and decreased levels of progesterone. Women may suffer symptoms ranging from severe cramping to cervical erosion, ovarian tumors, and increased risks of cervical cancer. Men continue to produce sperm at a rate of 50,000 per minute, but without a passage for exiting the testes, the sperm are either consumed by other cells or degenerate on their own. The resulting antigens can enter the bloodstream to produce antisperm auto-antibodies throughout the body. Over a period of 10 to 20 years, this autoimmunity may result in rheumatoid arthritis, atherosclerosis, diabetes, and other immunity disorders as well an increased risk for prostate cancer.

Most of the controversies surrounding the use of sterilization as a birth control method stem from its origins as a tool in the eugenics movement around the early 1900s. Thousands of prisoners and mental health patients were legally sterilized in the United States during the first half of the twentieth century. Advocates of compulsive sterilization argued that it was a technological solution to common social problems of habitual crime, vice, and mental illness. By the mid-1970s, such claims were rejected as gross violations of civil rights, and activists campaigned for policy safeguards that prevented anyone from being sterilized without their fully informed consent. Some of the provisions included 30-day waiting periods between when a woman consults with her doctor for sterilization and when she received the surgery. Sterilization for males did not receive as much scrutiny.

As with long-acting hormone contraceptives, the question of voluntariness remains a controversial issue related to sterilization. Feminists are divided on the issue, though all agree that involuntary sterilization violates fundamental civil rights. Some feminists argue that sterilization is one of many birth control options and that, as long as women choose it freely, it should be supported by public policy as strongly as any other method. Other feminists argue that women choose to permanently end their reproductive options only because they do not have adequate access to other, more reliable contraceptive methods and choose sterilization out of despair. These critics resist publicly supported sterilization programs unless they are accompanied by very strict safeguards. A key determinant of voluntariness among feminists is whether sterilization policies appear to be specifically targeted toward minority groups and the poor.

The question of voluntariness transcends the issue of public policy. Within families, there might be a debate over which spouse should give up his or her fertility. The decision to be sterilized carries with it increased risks of complications and higher probabilities for certain types of cancer for both men and women. Yet, statistically, three times as many women seek tubal ligations than men seeking vasectomies. Some of the reasons that might account for this disparity have little to do with actual research. They may include assumptions that women are ultimately responsible for procreation, fears that sterilized men may be more inclined to marital infidelity, or concerns that vasectomy may undermine male potency. Some feminists argue that men need to assume more responsibility in contraception. Other critics argue that the sterilization is naturally divisive to marriage and family and should be avoided for that reason.

Religious groups are also divided on the issue of sterilization. Up until 1930, all Christian denominations opposed deliberate sterilization as an immoral form of birth control because they viewed it as a form of self-mutilation. Christian denominations often refer to the body as a temple for the soul, and willful injury to natural functions of the body compromises the integrity of the human person, which integrates our physical body with the spirit of God. After the 1960s, however, following the introduction of the combination pill, Christian denominations also began to differ on the issue of sterilization. Some denominations argue that sterilization is yet another technological option given by God to mankind to aid in responsible family planning. Others, including the Catholic Church, continue to strongly oppose sterilization because it seeks to avoid the consequences of moral choices.

As with the division between natural and artificial contraceptives, the issues and controversies related to sterilization involve a complex array of considerations ranging from civil rights to moral discernment.

FORCED STERILIZATION AS SOCIAL REFORM?

Up until the nineteenth century, scientists believed any interference with the vans deferens would result in the equivalence of castration (referred to at the time as "unsexing"). In 1823, a British researcher, Ashley Cooper, discovered that vasectomy in dogs did not stop the production of sperm or the dog's coital activity. That same year, a London doctor, James Blundell, described a procedure by which a woman's fallopian tubes could be cut during a caesarean operation and end future pregnancies.

Neither Cooper nor Blundell attempted these procedures on humans, and it was not until 1881 that S. S. Lungren of Ohio attempted the first tubal ligation and 1891 before the procedure was performed with reliable results. The first vasectomy was performed in Sweden by H. D. Lennander as a therapy for prostate disease in 1897 and was not performed for purposes of birth control until a Chicago doctor, A. J. Ochsner, brought the procedure to the United States later that year. The following year, Ochsner published a paper that touted vasectomies as the ultimate solution to crime control and racial degeneracy. By 1899, sterilization became the most popular tool among eugenicists for eradicating such social problems as mental illness, habitual criminals, addiction to vice, and poverty.

Beginning in 1899, Dr. Harry Sharp of the Indiana State Reformatory at Jeffersonville performed several hundred vasectomies on inmates over the period of several years. He believed that he could best reform inmates as productive members of society by removing their excessive sexual impulses through vasectomies. In part, this view stemmed from the earlier (albeit refuted) association between vasectomy and castration. Reports of his activities spread throughout the criminal justice community, and sterilization was touted as a major innovation in prison reform.

Initially, Sharp received consent from the inmates before operating, but by 1907 the Indiana legislature passed a law that allowed him to sterilize inmates without their permission. The object of these laws was to prevent the insane, feebleminded, and habitual criminals from reproducing and potentially passing on their defective genes. Similar eugenic sterilization laws were passed in Washington, California, and 24 other states between 1909 and 1931. They were largely unquestioned until a Virginia family filed suit against the Virginia State Colony for Epileptics and Feeble Minded in 1924 in an attempt to prevent 18-year-old Carrie Buck from being sterilized against her will. The case went to the Supreme Court, which upheld the Virginia law. In the opinion, Justice Oliver Wendell Holmes concluded that "three generations of imbeciles are enough." The *Buck v. Bell* (1927) decision affirmed the constitutionality of involuntary sterilization for inmates under state care.

Eugenic sterilization laws remained actively enforced until after World War II, when public opinion on eugenics radically changed. The association with Hitler killed overt public support for eugenics programs in the United States. Enforcement of the sterilization laws declined significantly by the 1960s, and by the 1970s most state laws had been repealed. Beginning in the 1980s, the American Civil Liberties Union filed lawsuits in each state seeking compensation from the government's role in violating the civil rights of those who were forcibly sterilized between 1927 and 1974.

CONCLUSION

As Alan Guttmacher noted in the 1960s, some form of birth control has been used by societies around the globe for thousands of years. But the explosion in the number of artificial birth control alternatives really belongs to the twentieth century. When the only options were pessaries and condoms, the debate over birth control was more unidimensional. As the industrial revolution and its technological innovations led to IUDs and hormonal-based contraceptives, the debate assumed new dimensions. And now, in the twenty-first century, the availability of new streams of communication has added one more layer of debate. No discussion of the issues and controversies surrounding birth control can be complete without fully understanding the type of birth control method and the context in which it is used.

Despite the prevalence of birth control use in American society, the type and extent of public support for contraceptives remains very controversial. The root of all debate over birth control rests in the various presuppositions of moral order and natural law. At this level, there is little room for compromise and little hope for widespread public consensus. For the sake of policymakers who need to find some broad agreement, most debates avoid questions of universal principles and focus instead on specific questions of access, health, and propriety. At the level of public debate, the wide spectrum of moral assumptions can be more easily categorized into more manageable policy questions. Chapters 4 through 6 consider the following categories:

- **Health:** What are the short-term and long-term effects of particular birth control methods? To what extent should the government regulate these methods, and how should the public be best informed to make their own decisions? When do the needs of public health outweigh the freedom of individual choice? How does birth control impact the physical and psychological health of individual families?
- **Consumer Protection:** To what extent should birth control be debated in the public forum? What role does private industry play in influencing matters of public and private health? What responsibility does industry have in protecting the physical, psychological, and moral health of their customers? To what extent should the government regulate commercial advertising for the physical, psychological, and moral health of the public?
- **Public Funding:** How much money should state and federal government spend on birth control? Are moral and religious divisions relevant considerations in matters of public health and civil rights? Should the United States promote birth control as a foreign policy initiative?
- **Voluntariness:** Does government support of particular birth control methods interfere with individual freedom to refuse? Are certain kinds of contraceptives more likely than others to interfere with individual freedom? Should public policy regulate the extent to which private organizations can promote contraceptive use? To what degree can cultural pressures undermine individual freedom to use or refrain from using certain birth control methods?
- **Civil Rights:** To what extent is birth control a constitutionally protected right? How should the government guarantee access to birth control and for which methods? How can government policies safeguard the rights of minority populations while still serving the physical and moral health needs of the majority?

- **Gender Equity:** With whom should responsibility for birth control most rest: men or women? To what extent should spousal prerogatives determine family planning options? Should the government regulate conditions to promote particular priorities for male or female prerogatives over birth control options?
- **Age Appropriateness:** At what age can an individual intelligently and voluntarily decide on matters of birth control? To what extent should government policy guarantee the right of parents to protect their children from exposure to questions of human sexuality and birth control options? Does industry have a responsibility to safeguard children from their aggressive marketing techniques?

Broad consensus on particular public policy decisions remains rare, but compromises can be reached. Each theme triggers different debates among various groups, depending on their ideological presuppositions, and no single ideology enjoys dominant public support. Over the past 200 years, a number of ideological positions have emerged in reaction to technological and sociological changes in American history. Some of the positions form natural alliances with others, and others are inherently antagonistic. But most of these positions remain separate, and temporary coalitions of viewpoints often come together in response to specific policy questions. These coalitions usually dissolve when the particular issue goes away. In some cases, the splintered parts reform into new coalitions for new questions—and opponents in one instance may be allied in another. Thorough understanding of each unique ideological presumption relative to birth control is necessary to better understand these dynamic shifts in American political culture. The next two chapters consider those historic positions that still have an impact on public policy debates today.

CHAPTER 2

History of Birth Control— From the American Revolution to World War II

Contraceptives have been present in human societies for thousands of years, but with few exceptions their usage remained limited to the margins of society. The history of their use in the United States shows a similar pattern. At the start of American history, contraceptives were viewed as both a political and a moral evil. People might use them privately, but very few would publicly admit to it. Contraceptives were linked too strongly to immorality and obscenity for it to be publicly recognized or even discussed.

By the turn of the twentieth century, these views had begun to change. Mostly, it was in reaction to the success of the industrial revolution and the public's newfound willingness to apply scientific methods to solve social problems. Rapid changes in American demographics led to a reappraisal of cultural priorities. Most of the ideals of the late 1800s carried over to the early 1900s but with a slightly different emphasis.

The impact of World War I intensified some of the technological changes and contributed to some social anxiety about American identity. The nation strongly endorsed two major social reforms with the passage of the Eighteenth and Nineteenth Amendments to the U.S. Constitution, but woman suffrage and prohibition did not imply full consensus on other matters of public morality. Advocates for the legalization of contraceptives and birth control education successfully used the postwar ambiguity to push for a public debate on the subject.

On the eve of World War II, most churches had considered the morality of contraceptives but had not achieved a consensus. The issue was brought to the public forum, but no clear consensus was achieved. Public display and advertisement of contraceptives remained illegal in most states, but medical prescription was legalized on the federal level, and private use increased significantly. Contraception was no longer restricted to the margins of society, but neither was it fully embraced as a mainstream medical technology. Yet this minor shift in public policy represented a revolutionary change in the ideological approach to birth control. To understand the scope of these changes, it is necessary to look more closely at the nineteenth-century worldview.

REPUBLICAN MOTHERHOOD

Prior to the nineteenth century, government policy in Europe and the United States opposed contraception on principle because it weakened the nation's resources. Population was included among cultivable land, navigable ports, mineral supplies, and military technology as key indicators of national wealth. Specific policies limiting family size were unknown, and the social culture promoted fecundity as an end in itself. Evidence of contraceptive practices left by private writings of doctors, herbalists, and midwifes indicate that some women infrequently sought to avoid or terminate their pregnancy. But the scarcity of such accounts suggests that these practices were followed discreetly, or secretly, out of fear of public disapproval (legal or otherwise).

Around the time of the revolution, Americans placed special value on motherhood because it reinforced both spiritual and political priorities of the new democracy. Thomas Jefferson wrote that "all men were created equal, and were endowed by the Creator with certain unalienable rights . . . ," thereby placing the burden of government on the shoulders of the American people. Democracy requires an educated public. At the time, public education was still in its infancy, and most primary schooling occurred in the home. The responsibility fell to mothers to provide their children with the necessary tools to be intelligent leaders of the future. This role of motherhood was more than a social duty—it rose to the level of a spiritual obligation. God created the natural order of humanity to exercise their rights of "life, liberty, and the pursuit of happiness," so failure to prepare the next generation to assume those responsibilities amounted to a failure to discharge a vocation under God. Historians refer to this ideal as **Republican Motherhood**, and it helps to explain why women were often held up as models of excellence and purity during the eighteenth and nineteenth centuries.

Feminist historians contend that the ideal of Republican Motherhood was a double-edge sword. It may have forced men to honor women as models of purity, but in so doing it also barred them from engaging in public affairs outside the home because such activities might corrupt their sensitive natures. The ideal also forced women to accept and embrace motherhood whether they wanted to or not. The alternative ideal of a professional woman, free from familial obligations, was foreign to nineteenth-century America. In this context, contraception violated not only traditional civic values of national wealth through population growth but also the divine mission of American exceptionalism. A woman's primary job was to raise and nurture the young, and any attempt to sabotage or avoid that obligation was regarded either as a personal failure or as a moral affront. Whether or not explicit laws existed to forbid the practice, contraception was viewed as an act of deviancy that respectable people avoided.

SOCIAL SCIENCE REFORM

The first public calls to reconsider the inherent value of large families and uninhibited reproduction came from a small group of intellectuals trying to apply scientific principles to social planning. In 1798, political economist Thomas Malthus became alarmed by what he perceived as declining living conditions associated with the rapidly growing cities in England, especially London. England was experiencing an industrial revolution, and a large percentage of its population was moving from a rural to a more urbanized lifestyle. Malthus was born and raised on a country estate and viewed the cramped conditions of the working poor in London as deplorable, blaming the problem on increasing population densities. In his famous work *An Essay on the Principles of Population*, Malthus compared the conditions of urban dwellers to the plight of animals in their natural environment. He observed that if all the offspring of a species were allowed to reach maturity, they would outstrip its food supply in a matter of generations. In the wild, disease and predation serve as natural checks against this overpopulation. Malthus concluded that human populations work in the same fashion and are directly tied to the level of available resources. When times are plentiful, the population increases. But when resources become scarce, the population naturally falls through famine and disease.

Malthus was not proposing that populations be held in check; instead, he was arguing in support of more proactive domestic policies to encourage greater production of resources. Malthus viewed food supply, not population, as the active variable. Nevertheless, his theories had tremendous influence on later social scientists who built off of Malthus's conclusions in a variety of ways. Some philosophers began devising "perfect societies" that balanced resource supplies and population demands, including the French utopian socialists Henri de Saint-Simon and Charles Fourier and Scottish businessmen Robert Owen and Jeremy Bentham, the latter of whom actually invested their own money to build a utopian community in Indiana called New Harmony. These and other philosopher-based social scientists examined human society in the same way that a biologist might examine plants and animals. Human conception became one of many variables that could be manipulated to achieve some social or political ideal.

In 1859, another intellectual child of Thomas Malthus, Charles Darwin, published *The Origin of the Species*, which postulated that animal life evolved over the course of millennia. He followed it up in 1871 with *The Descent of Man*, which suggested that humans arose from a similar process. This theory of evolution is most known for its role in questioning biblical accounts of human creation. In terms of birth control, Darwin was far more influential in further opening the door for later intellectuals to reexamine human life apart from its teleology. Like Malthus's theory of overpopulation, the theory of evolution spawned numerous ideologies that were only tangentially connected to biology and natural science.

For some social scientists, evolution provided a missing link for explaining natural solutions to age-old social problems such as poverty, disease, criminal behavior, and mental illness. Since ancient times, aristocratic ideology relied on generalized theories of heredity to explain why certain families were favored over others. It believed that bloodlines held imperceptible qualities that set the greater families apart from the commoners. Darwin's theories provided a new framework for explaining these social differences in ways that appeared quite modern and intellectually objective. In 1869, a cousin of Darwin, Francis Galton, used statistical methodology to study the hereditary causes for genius and greatness in *Hereditary Genius*. He focused special interest on the tension between the hereditary forces that predispose some people toward great (or corrupt) futures and the nurturing influences of family upbringing that either promoted or counteracted those natural tendencies. Galton coined the phrase "Nature versus Nurture" to describe this tension and spent years collating the family histories of great figures in history to identify the extent to which one persons' greatness (or failure) was reflected in the greatness (or failure) of their relatives. In 1883, Galton published *Inquiries into Human Faculty and Its Development* to introduce the scientific theory of **eugenics**, which combined elements of Malthus, Darwin, and the utopian socialists to argue that a more perfect human race

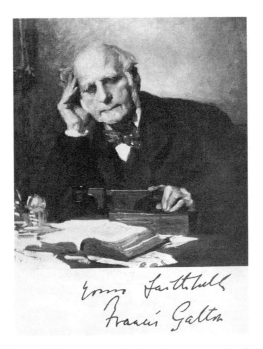

Great Britain's Francis Galton was a nineteenth-century scientist and anthropologist whose achievements spanned an incredible variety of fields and disciplines. He is best known as the inventor of the science of eugenics. (Library of Congress)

could be crafted from careful manipulation of human breeding. Outside of academics, Galton strongly encouraged laws in England to promote marriages between high-ranking families and penalties for the "irresponsible breeding" among the lesser ranks.

The theory of eugenics played an enormous role in the history of birth control policy in the United States. Prior to the 1860s, the few manuals for contraception published in France fell into one of two categories: spurious scientific texts used to cover prurient interests or genuinely practical texts intended to be given (discreetly) to young couples by doctors in the privacy of their office. Public distribution of these manuals, regardless of which kind they were, was viewed as indecent—akin to distributing pornography. To some extent, this view grew out of the reality that many of these texts were, in fact, prurient by intention. Yet beyond that evidence, any frank discussion of sexuality was seen as inappropriate for the public square. In 1832, Charles Knowlton was convicted of obscenity three times in Massachusetts, fined $50, and forced to serve three months of hard labor for publishing *The Fruits of Philosophy*, which detailed various methods of contraception. Knowlton was a self-described "freethinker" and promoted birth control as a natural advance of modern science. There were no laws explicitly forbidding the publication of birth control manuals, but the courts repeatedly applied existing laws against obscenity to Knowlton's case because, according to the communities of the 1830s, there was no difference between the two types of materials.

Richard Carlile published *What Is Love?* in 1826. It was the first English-language pamphlet on birth control. He was known for publishing many controversial works and was imprisoned throughout his life on various charges of blasphemy, libel, and sedition. Whether Carlile sincerely promoted birth control, whether he was simply testing the boundaries of England's censorship laws, or whether he used the topic as a more scientific cover for more prurient purposes is unclear.

Around the same time that Carlile published his book, a Scottish socialist named Robert Dale Owen came to the United States and became a newspaper editor in New York. In 1830, he wrote *Moral Physiology*, which became the first book on birth control published in the United States. The following year, his friend, Dr. Charles Knowlton of Massachusetts, published a more extensive book on the subject titled *The Fruits of Philosophy* (1831). Both Owen and Knowlton framed their books around Thomas Malthus's theories of overpopulation, which laid the basis for later advocates of birth control education for more than a century.

Malthus was still alive when Carlile, Owen, and Knowlton published their works, but he was not in agreement with their reinterpretation or their methods. Malthus, an Anglican curate (similar to a priest), opposed arguments advocating birth control as the deliberate "check" on population. Instead, he recommended that couples delay marriage until later in life, thereby limiting the number of children without relying any unnatural methods.

Malthus also opposed efforts to promote "preventive checks" on population, ideas that later developed into the eugenics movement. As Malthus warned, such programs would condemn "all the bad specimens to celibacy." As a minister, Malthus hoped that the fear of overpopulation would reinforce existing moral sanctions against sexual relations outside of marriage. His political agenda was focused more on encouraging government support for urban health and welfare programs in increasingly dense urban populations.

By contrast to Malthus, both Carlile and Knowlton were avowed atheists. Although Knowlton strongly endorsed Malthus's theory of pending overpopulation, he objected to religious-based solutions and advocated more proactive—even radical—proposals for dealing with it. In the United States, Knowlton and other "freethinkers" translated Malthus's theories into a political ideology. A series of birth control manuals came out in the decades that followed, and almost all of them point first to Malthus and the dangers of overpopulation. It is unlikely that Malthus would have found much sympathy with most of those later authors. For more information on this subject, check out selections from Knowlton and E. B. Foote in Section III.

After the 1860s, there was a shift in tone used in the science-based birth control manuals. Rather than providing a voluntary alternative for young couples who may want to delay conception, the new manuals tended to read like social polemics that argued for increasing conceptive education in order to protect society from irresponsible breeding. In 1886, E. B. Foote argued that society was plagued by four "radical evils," which he listed as ignorance, reckless propagation, evil hereditary influence, and overpopulation in his book *Radical Remedies in Social Science* (also titled *Borning Better Babies through Regulating Reproduction by Controlling Conception*). After quoting Thomas Malthus and Herbert Spencer, Foote reduced all the problems of modern society down to general ignorance of how reckless propagation, overpopulation, and evil hereditary are responsible for all vice, crime, mental illness, and other human problems. His radical remedy, therefore, was to promote a proactive education program to ensure that "every man and woman at the age of puberty shall know enough, and be religiously inclined to guard against crippling himself or herself, the family of society, by indulging in vice of any kind, and in particular that of reckless propagation." Foote's argument was not unique. It represented a trend among certain social scientists who viewed birth control less as a matter of private family planning and more as a vehicle for radical social reform. Some argued that "responsible propagation" could cure poverty by reducing the number of poor workers and increase genius and greatness by promoting desirable matches between the better classes. Although this association with radical social reform promoted wider education of contraception, it also triggered a significant reaction among more traditional reformers who still viewed vice and moral corruption as the primary cause for social evil.

TEMPERANCE AND PURITY MOVEMENTS

In part, the success of contraception education as a vehicle for radical reform grew out of the social environment of the 1880s to 1910s that witnessed unprecedented changes as a result of industrialization. Like Malthus reacting to the exploding urbanization of London, certain concerned Americans reacted to the decline of agriculture as the primary source of their prosperity, the rapid mechanization of labor, the birth of giant multistate corporations holding greater wealth than most state governments, the constant influx of immigrants looking for work in the new economy, and the rise of densely populated urban centers intent on housing them all together. Eugenicists were not alone in their call for proactive action to solve rising crime rates, political machines, sanitation problems, and concentrated ignorance that these urban environments seemed to create. Marxists, socialists, anarchists, freethinkers, free lovers, and a host of others could be counted as "liberals" reacting positively and negatively to industrialization. The number of "radical remedies" easily kept pace with the number of technological innovations that fueled the rapid changes.

In the midst of the urbanization, immigration, and mechanization that followed American industrialization, another group of more traditional moral reformers coalesced under the banner of **temperance** and served as a major counterpoint to the radical options. Tracing their authority back to America's long religious traditions, these moral reformers blamed the anonymity of dense populations for creating a lax moral environment that allowed vice and corruption to arise. Industrialization was not the problem; rather, individual moral character was the problem, and urban centers did little to protect its proper development. The first temperance groups arose shortly after the American Revolution, when local towns outlawed or limited the sale of alcohol in order to encourage the sobriety of the electorate. During the Second Great Awakening in the 1820s, the American Temperance Society was formed to promote the moral health of American society through clean and sober living. This organization, however, was comprised of hundreds of very small groups focused on the specific conditions of morality in their local towns or communities and had little national coordination.

Although temperance is often associated with laws banning or limiting the sale of alcohol, the movement was initially led by fiery preachers who always included larger principles of self-restraint and moral discipline. Alcohol was included among other vices, such as tobacco, gambling, and prostitution, all of which undermined the home and corrupted the innocence of youth. During the 1850s until the Civil War, the temperance movement joined other moral reform groups to narrow their focus more specifically on solving the problem of slavery and addressing obvious civil rights abuses. After the war and after abolition ceased to be an issue, the temperance movement reemerged, this time as a grassroots reaction to the increasingly public calls for more "radical remedies" to solve social problems, especially those calling for more explicit education of contraceptive practices. Addiction to alcohol and narcotics remained a major issue for temperance movements, but during the 1870s and 1880s, moral continence and individual purity were often more important.

In 1874, Francis Willard, a former president of Evanston College for Ladies, launched a 50-day lecture tour promoting the temperance movement and its ideals of individual self-restraint. She also promoted woman suffrage as a necessary step in ensuring the protection of the home. She and others helped form the Women's Christian Temperance Union (WCTU) and eventually served as its president from 1879 to her death in 1898. The mission of the WCTU was to educate the public on the dangers posed by vice, alcoholism, and addiction to the family home. Alcohol, vice, and other impurities all threatened families, and women needed to be politically active in order to protect their homes.

The WCTU grew very quickly and expanded into several distinct bureaus. The most publicized arm was the Speakers Bureau, which included dozens of clergymen, women, and other reform leaders who traveled across the country to speak to local organizations on a variety of topics ranging from moral purity, antivice, and woman suffrage. The Scientific Temperance Federation was a WCTU bureau charged with using the tools of modern science in order to gather statistics and other quantifiable evidence showing the effect of alcohol, tobacco, and other vices on the family and child welfare. The Education Bureau published thousands of pamphlets and school packets to encourage purity pledges among school-age children. These pledges vowed not only abstinence from alcohol but also abstinence and avoidance of other behaviors that threatened individual morality (sexual and otherwise). Students who signed the pledge wore specially knotted white ribbons to show their commitment to a temperate life.

The WCTU and complementary temperance and purity movements resulted not only in the introduction of numerous laws limiting or banning the sale of alcohol and tobacco but also in the passage of other purity laws, including raising the age of consent (which in some states was set at 10 or 12 years), enforcement of more severe penalties for molestation (child rape), and the legal censorship of pornography and indecency. The WCTU's Department for the Promotion of Purity in Literature and Art was formed in 1883, and by 1900 there were 168,000 active members enrolled in 7,000 local chapters of the WCTU throughout the country.

COMSTOCK AND CONTRACEPTION

During this same time, Anthony Comstock gained public attention in New York City by leading raids on Manhattan book sellers who sold erotic and pornographic fiction. He gained so much public support that leaders within the New York YMCA asked Comstock to lead the New York Society of the Suppression of Vice. Within a year, in 1873, Comstock lobbied the U.S. Congress to pass a national law prohibiting the use of mails for indecent materials. He argued that "social vice and national decay stand to each other as parent to child, cause to consequence, fountain to

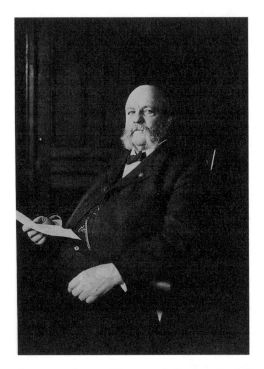

Anthony Comstock was such a well-known defender of public morality in the United States around the turn of the nineteenth century that his name became synonymous with moralistic censorship. (Library of Congress)

stream, the one begetting, the other begotten." Comstock targeted pornography and other indecent materials because it perverted the imagination of young people, which, he believed, affixed a black stain on a child's conscience, rendering it "seared and silenced." This purity movement operated in parallel with the temperance movement.

With broad public support, Congress passed the **Comstock Law** of 1873, which made it a felony to "sell or lend, or give away, or in any manner exhibit, or ... publish or offer to publish in any manner, or ... have in [one's possession], for any purpose or purposes, any obscene book, pamphlet, paper, writing, advertisement, circular, print, picture, drawing or other representation, figure, or image on or of paper or other material, or any cast, instrument or other article of an immoral nature, or any drug or medicine, or any article what ever for the prevention of conception, or for causing unlawful abortion, or ... advertize same for sale." The primary purpose of the Comstock Law was to target pornography and other indecent materials. Contraception was included as a final clause and was grouped among the "instrument[s] or other article[s] of an immoral nature." In part, the clause was included to target those pseudopornographic books that tried to hide behind the category of "sex manuals." In part, the clause was also intended to provide some consumer protection against scam artists who promised cures for sterility or fecundity through quick-fix manuals that pretended to be scientific. The critical point was that under the Comstock Law contraception was not considered as either a medical or a scientific issue but solely as a moral issue.

The public sensitivity to indecency was particularly high during the time of the temperance and purity movements of 1870s, and the Comstock Law lent itself to very broad interpretations. After Congress passed the law, Anthony Comstock returned to New York to serve as its primary censor for the U.S. Post Office, authorized to inspect packages and prosecute those who sent "obscene, lewd, or lascivious" materials through the mail. Neither Congress nor Comstock could specifically quantify the definition of obscenity, so their decisions invited some controversy when literary figures such as D. H. Lawrence, Theodore Dreiser, and George Bernard Shaw were barred from publishing their materials because the subject matter was deemed offensive. For these and other decisions, Comstock drew criticism among the liberal social reformers who balked at the legal censorship. Nevertheless, for most of the nation, Comstock represented the official standard of decency and cleanliness in public communication during the last few decades of the 1800s.

As a result of the Comstock laws, all materials related to contraception were explicitly prohibited from being sent through the mails. Comstock and his public decency movement could not easily prevent the initial publication of these materials, but their exclusion from the mail system significantly curtailed distribution. In addition, a legal question remained about whether the Comstock Law could apply to doctors prescribing specific materials within the privacy of the medical office. At the time of its passage, in 1874, the issue did not arise because the primary concern was to prohibit pornographic books that were hiding behind the facade of medical instruction. Generations later, in 1936, a federal circuit court was asked reexamine the Comstock Law in *U.S. v. One Package of Japanese Pessaries*. The court concluded that the right and authority for dispensing contraceptive methods and devices lay solely with the medical community. After 60 years, the Second Circuit Court concluded that the federal Comstock Law was not meant to prevent importation, sale, or carriage of things "intelligently employed by conscientious and competent physicians for the purpose of saving life or promoting the well-being of their patients." The changes in cultural priorities from 1874 to 1936 were enormous. The most significant, though, was the shift in the public perception that initially viewed contraception as a moral issue that threatened public decency to the later view of birth control as a scientific tool used to protect families and public health.

THE PROGRESSIVE ERA

During the 30 years after the Civil War, the temperance movement had much greater public support than the few social scientists and radical reformers who were calling for unconditional embrace of scientific solutions. In part, the success of the temperance movement reflected public reaction to unsettling social changes brought about by the industrial revolution. The advocates behind the purity movement and the Comstock laws were not opposed to technological progress per se, but they were concerned by the lack of balance between scientific innovation and moral development.

The tide began to turn for the temperance movement around 1900. The industrial revolution was no longer new, and dense urban living conditions became the norm rather than the exception. More important, the growth of large corporations and heavy industry improved the standard of living for all sectors. Prices of manufactured goods fell, salaries increased, and a flood of time-saving inventions improved communication, transportation, and entertainment. Despite the rapid social changes, few could deny the fact that science brought many useful solutions.

Historians named the period from 1895 to 1915 the **Progressive Era** because almost all leading figures shared a broad faith in the nation's ability to continually progress through its industry and technological innovation. Ideological opponents still sharply disagreed about the proper method for solving social problems, but all sides generally agreed that with common effort and commitment, the nation could solve any problem. Politicians from both parties called themselves "Progressives" because they believed that experts could help state and local government become more professional and efficient, less corrupt and wasteful, and better able to solve urban issues, such as job safety, personal security, and public sanitation.

The temperance movement of the 1870s did not disappear, but it did shift its priorities. Rather than focusing on such abstract goals as individual moral restraint and protecting purity, the temperance movement focused on the one problem that most contributed to the worsening of the others: alcohol. After Francis Willard's death in 1898, the WCTU joined more closely with the Anti-Saloon League to refocus its attention mostly on scientific temperance, which used the statistical tools of social science to provide compelling arguments for the destructive impact of alcohol on family, its economic tolls on workplace and productivity, and its association with public corruption and political scandal. In this new manifestation, the temperance movement found much greater success. The omnipartisan Anti-Saloon League attracted supporters inside and outside of the church movement and eventually brought about passage of the Nineteenth Amendment, which prohibited the manufacture or sale of alcohol (Prohibition) from 1919 to 1934.

This shift in focus from generalized restraint to specific abstention from alcohol was significant for the history of contraception because it changed the conditions of the public debate. No longer strictly a moral issue, alcohol abuse became a scientific problem with a possible scientific solution. Political reformers could support the measure as a way to protect women and the family and to promote social evolution through more healthy living. They could also include the plank in their general platform of political reform regardless of their political party or religious affiliation. But in so doing, the temperance and purity movements also gave up their primary defense against other science-based reform measures, thereby opening the door for reconsiderations of contraception within the framework of science.

Direct discussions of sexual practices, even from a scientific framework, were still considered obscene and were still prohibited by most Comstock laws. Likewise, in most states, the use of contraceptive devices was still illegal under obscenity laws, but the enforcement of those laws began to fall precipitously by the 1910s and 1920s. In some urban centers, such as Boston or New York, radical reformers opened shops that sold contraception literature and devices with little worry of prosecution. Among those who had the means to procure them, the discreet use of pessaries and condoms became relatively common in urban centers, though open discussion about them was still not socially acceptable. It was during this time period and in one such shop that Margaret Sanger first entered into public notice.

SANGER, SCIENCE, AND RADICALISM

Margaret Higgins was born in Corning, New York, as one of 11 children in 1879. Her father was a stone carver and was described as a freethinker who supported the progressive issues of the times, including woman suffrage, free public education, progressive income taxes, and labor reform. There was no evidence of unusual deprivation as a child, but her mother died of tuberculosis and cervical cancer when Margaret was still in her teens. She left home to train as a nurse, and while at school she met and married an architect named William Sanger, who was very active in the Socialist Party and the radical bohemian culture of Greenwich Village in New York City.

Sanger first learned about contraception as a necessary component to "free love" (sex outside marriage), which she experimented with in the radical community. It was not until she began working as a nurse among the poor working mothers of New York City's Lower East Side that Sanger began promoting contraception as a tool for married couples. Sanger concluded that one of the major reasons for "misery among workers" was uncontrolled pregnancies and too many mouths to feed. After splitting from her husband, Sanger started her own campaign promoting contraception as a form of social reform and launched a magazine dedicated to the subject titled *The Woman Rebel—No Gods, No Masters*. Sanger is credited with coining the term "birth control," but she initially limited her discussion of the subject to generalities, focusing primarily on the connection between poverty, disease, and large families.

One anecdote that Sanger often repeated in her speeches was about her visit to the apartment of a Jewish immigrant named Sadie Sachs, who suffered from complications from a self-induced abortion. Sanger claimed that Sachs asked a doctor for help but was told simply to abstain from sexual intercourse. A few months later, Sachs was found dead after trying to use a coat hanger to induce another abortion. There is no historical evidence for the story, but the image of the cold indifference of a doctor denying contraceptive information resulting in a woman's death was a powerful rhetorical tool. Sanger used the story repeatedly during the 1920s to promote legalization of contraception. Later, advocates from Planned Parenthood used a similar version of the same story during the 1960s to promote legalization of abortion. The importance of the story is that it helped Sanger link contraception to women's rights—a complete reversal from the temperance and purity movements a generation earlier, which also promoted the protection of women to justify their prohibition of contraception and other indecent materials.

Sanger's opposition to the temperance and purity movements was not unique. A segment of social scientists had become increasingly antagonistic to the influence of religious morality on both academia and public policy. The Comstock Law prohibited the publication and dissemination of obscene materials, but that had little effect on professors and researchers in the newly emerging fields of sociology and psychology. One female professor at Wellesley, Mary Roberts Smith, conducted a survey on the sexual attitudes of normal women in 1890. She concluded that her sample (women from the upper/middle class) wanted better access to contraceptive information and devices. Smith further concluded that many women suffered from "sex anxiety" because they feared that sexual activity would lead to pregnancy, inadvertently limiting their independence outside a family home. Although Sigmund Freud never published on the issue of contraception, his theory of psychosexual development were being promulgated at the same time as Smith's research and was completely compatible with the conclusions. Many researchers in the United States and Europe had begun to examine sexuality as a scientific issue outside the domains of morality. In practice, however, these scholars were not read much outside the tight circle of academia, and thus even though their research dealt with human production, they did so in a strictly scientific manner, triggering little concern from the Comstock officials.

NEO-MALTHUSIANS VERSUS EUGENICS

Most of the academics who looked into contraception did so with the purpose of population control and/or eugenics. Just prior to World War I, a group of social scientists identified collectively as "neo-Malthusians" began to argue that the conflict was a natural result of overpopulation and resource scarcity. Applying Malthus to the twentieth century, they argued that the industrialized nations were forced into competitive struggles over resources, and fighting was the inevitable result. Even though Malthus rejected contraception as a solution in his 1798 essay, they claimed that he would have recommended it as a technological innovation necessary to avoid repeated world wars for the future. Their debates, however, had much less political influence than their eugenics-based colleagues.

Eugenicists generally opposed contraception because they argued that only the educated "well-bred" classes would be sensible enough to use it and that the "dependent" classes would ignore it. Improper use of contraception might result in "race suicide"—a term used by eugenicists as a warning to depict the consequences of allowing the dependent classes to thrive while the well-bred classes declined. As one eugenicist explained, "Defectives of the lower types do not greatly limit sex indulgence by the fear of having children, nor do they resort to artificial means to prevent conception."

Eugenics-based social scientists did support sterilization, and they launched a strong lobbying campaign to change state laws to permit involuntary sterilization of certain criminals and others deemed mentally unstable. The American Eugenics Society did not officially form until 1926, but arguments that preceded it were quite common among social scientists, especially within the field of sociology. Between 1905 and 1922, there were 30 bills passed in 18 states, resulting in the involuntary sterilizations of thousands of inmates in prisons and mental health facilities.

The Supreme Court ruled in *Buck v. Bell* (1927) that states could legally enact laws to forcibly sterilize people deemed "unfit" for reproduction. In his decision, Justice Oliver Wendell Holmes argued, "It is better for all the world, if instead of waiting to execute degenerate offspring for crime, or to let them starve for their imbecility, society can prevent those who are manifestly unfit from continuing their kind. The principle that sustains compulsory vaccination is broad enough to cover cutting the Fallopian tubes."

After World War II exposed the horrors of Adolf Hitler's death camps, the academic support for eugenics disappeared very quickly. Hitler's National Socialist (Nazi) Party used race-based arguments and other racial theories to divide people among the "well bred" (Aryans) and the "undesirable" (non-Aryans). The dictatorship sterilized more than 2 million women in Germany's Rassenhygiene (race hygiene) program. Later, during a three-year period between 1942 and 1945, the German Reich exterminated nearly 10 million "undesirables" in an effort to further "cleanse" German society.

After the war ended and the extent of death and destruction was revealed, no scientist wanted to be associated with the atrocious brutality of Nazism. The formal eugenics movement died with the war. The Supreme Court initiated the process with *Skinner v. Oklahoma* (1942), which ruled that states could not impose sterilization as a criminal penalty. By the 1960s, most states had ended the practice of forcibly sterilizing the "incorrigible" and "feebleminded." Nevertheless, the controversy of forcible sterilization resurfaced again in the 1980s after the invention of long-acting contraceptives.

The postwar history for neo-Malthusian ideology was much different. The concern for overpopulation intensified during the Cold War, as some social scientists made the argument that the poverty of Third World nations made them more susceptible to communist insurrections. By the 1960s, the ecology movement shifted focus away from strictly political or economic concerns to concentrate more on environmental issues. The nature of Malthusian ideology had changed drastically between proponents of the 1910s, just as it had from that originally articulated by Thomas Malthus himself in the 1790s. Rather than predicting dire consequences for humanity as overpopulation led to unavoidable natural checks (such as famine, disease, and war), the new "deep ecology" warned of the dire consequences that overpopulation posed to the nonhuman life forms. The Malthusian theory in its many various ideological forms is still common in the twenty-first century. Dozens of associations organized to address Malthusian concerns currently exist, including Population Action International (established in 1965), Zero Population Growth (now Population Connection, established in 1968), Negative Population Growth (established in 1972), the Voluntary Human Extinction Movement (established in 1996), and the International Society of Malthus (established in 1997).

In contrast to the discussions of eugenics and social engineering held by academicians, Sanger operated outside the classroom setting. She directly targeted the institutions of temperance and moral purity that dominated mainstream society during the late 1800s. In the third issue of *The Woman Rebel*, Sanger described the YMCA and YWCA as "brothels of the spirit and morgues of Freedom!" She also condemned the Catholic Church for subjugating women by turning them into "mere incubators." During her early writing, Sanger's views were more strongly defined by tactics of the radical labor movement, which included inflammatory rhetoric and deliberate defiance of legal authority when it ran counter to the movement. At the same time, Sanger also added a radical tone to the more academic-based eugenics movement. In the same article, Sanger defined birth control as "nothing more or less than the facilitation of the process of weeding out the unfit [and] of preventing the birth of defectives. . . . If we are to make racial progress, this development of womanhood must precede motherhood in every individual woman. Then and then only can the mother cease to be an incubator and be a mother indeed. Then only can she transmit to her sons and daughters the qualities which make strong individuals and, collectively, a strong race." After a single year in 1914, Sanger's publications, combined with the public speeches and agitation, triggered notice from the usually lax attention of the Comstock Law enforcers. Faced with multiple charges of Comstock violations as well as a charge of inciting assassination (Sanger called for the assassination of John D. Rockefeller in her first issue of *The Woman Rebel*), Sanger avoided prosecution by fleeing to England, where she remained for most of 1915.

When she returned to the United States in 1916, Sanger dedicated herself fully to the cause of promoting birth control. While visiting a Dutch clinic, she became convinced that diaphragms were the most effective contraceptive device and managed to smuggle some samples on her return. For years, she lobbied Congress to ease trading restrictions to permit diaphragms as a medical device. Sanger also opened a birth control clinic in the Brownsville section of Brooklyn, New York, in 1917 and was arrested on obscenity charges a week later. She launched another magazine called *Birth Control Review* and organized a new organization called the American Birth Control League in 1921. Although she was arrested on several occasions during her early career, Sanger's work was relatively unhindered during the 1920s. During most of the 1910s and early 1920s, Sanger was viewed as a radical socialist, but she was nevertheless successful in shifting the debate away from obscenity and toward a more scientific basis for family planning.

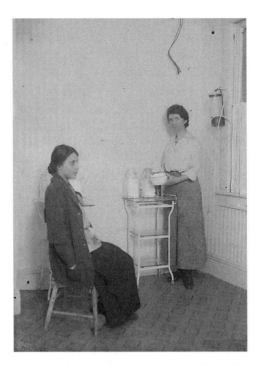

Margaret Sanger and Fania Mindell in the Brownsville Clinic, October 1916.
(Courtesy of the George Grantham Bain Collection, Library of Congress)

THE TOWN HALL RAID

On November 13, 1921, Sanger was scheduled to speak at the New
York City Town Hall on the subject of "Birth Control: Is It Moral?"
Accompanying her was Harold Cox and Mary Winsor. Cox was the editor
of an English newspaper and a member of the British Parliament. Mary
Winsor was an American actress who had been active in the woman suffrage movement. Shortly before Sanger was ready to take the stage, a
group of police officers arrived to say that they would not be allowed to
speak. They proceeded to lock the doors and escort the speakers from
the stage. As the three were being taken out, the crowd began to chant,
"Defy them! Defy them!" at which point Sanger attempted to retake the
stage. She and the others were then arrested. As she was leaving, Sanger
is quoted as having said, "We have reason to believe that this meeting
was closed by the influence of the Catholic Church." Archbishop Patrick
Hayes had been invited to the function, and though he had not attended,
he sent his secretary, Monsignor Joseph Dineen, in his stead. Both the

monsignor and the bishop denied having any hand in alerting the police. Later, Sanger reported in her *Birth Control Review* that the Catholic archbishop of New York, Patrick Hayes, was responsible for ordering the police to stop the meeting.

Initially, the local press was supportive of the police action. After the war and the world's first successful communist revolution in Russia, radicals in the United States became increasingly active—and in some cases increasingly violent. Sanger's association as a radical socialist prompted the *New York Times* to write an editorial praising the efforts of the police in cracking down on what they perceived to be radical activists and reaffirming the traditional view that voluntary parenthood was not suitable for public discussion. A month later, Archbishop Hayes issued a pastoral letter to be read at all Sunday masses. It was also published by the *New York Times*. Hayes repeated the Church's condemnation of contraception from religious and moral standpoints, arguing that children were a blessing from God and that any effort to prevent childbirth was akin to refusing God's blessings. Echoing the arguments made by leaders of the temperance and purity movements a generation earlier, Hayes further asked all Catholics to protect their homes by preventing contraceptives and contraceptive literature from having any contact with their home and family. The letter did not make any mention of the Town Hall arrests, nor did it mention Sanger or her organization.

The *New York Times* unwittingly brought the issue of contraception to the public forum. Sanger wrote a rebuttal to the archbishop's pastoral letter and reached a significantly larger audience than she ever could have through her speeches and private magazine. Rather than addressing the morality of contraception directly, Sanger chose to direct attention to the Catholic Church and its non-American origins. While recognizing the Church's right to instruct its own members on moral lessons, Sanger criticized "attempts to make these ideas legislative acts and enforce its opinions and code of morals upon the Protestant members of this country, then I do consider its attempt an interference with the principle of this democracy, and I have a right to protest."

The archbishop responded in an editorial, again through the *New York Times*, condemning Sanger's lack of respect for the law and her willingness to be arrested to further her political goal. His goal was to bring public attention back to Sanger's radicalism, to which the *New York Times* and other postwar politicians were especially sensitive. However, Sanger's initial rebuttal had tapped into another postwar legacy, one that proved to have a more enduring impact. Within months, Sanger managed to elicit criticism and in some cases condemnation for the police action, opening the way for tacit approval of her activism.

The public sentiment in 1921 reflected a complex mix of emotions. The United States had earlier tipped the balance in favor of the Allies and helped win the war. But in so doing, it also abandoned a long isolationist tradition of staying out of European affairs. President Woodrow Wilson had promised that American involvement would bring about a new world order based on the rule of international law. Unfortunately, many Americans viewed the Treaty of Versailles as little more than a reaffirmation of the British and French empires, and the U.S. Congress rejected it not once but twice. The feeling of disillusionment and betrayal that followed manifested itself in a variety of ways. Some reformers sought a recommitment to America's moral exceptionalism, while others looked for more practical law enforcement in America's burgeoning cities, and some experimented with the sensual nightlife of the jazz clubs, while still others turned to radicalism.

The 1920 presidential election was won by Harding's pledge to "return to normalcy." Both guaranteeing women the right to vote and outlawing the sale and manufacture of alcohol were reform measures promoted by the temperance movements of the past century. Part of the momentum for passing two constitutional amendments in rapid succession was due to a national pressure to reclaim American identity after the war.

For others, the drive to restore American moral order manifested itself in intense nativism, including membership in the Ku Klux Klan. The group reorganized itself during the war with a new mission of protecting American values against foreign corruption, especially from Catholics, Jews, and labor radicals. In Indiana alone, the Klan boasted a membership of 118,000—about a quarter of the adult male population. Aside from the strong anti-Catholicism, the Klan was also strongly in favor of Prohibition and promised to enforce the law with or without police support. The Klan remained a small minority in American politics and suffered its own series of scandals in 1928, resulting in its eventual collapse. Nevertheless, there were millions of other Americans who shared similar forms of undefined anxiety about the nation's cultural identity.

To some extent, it was this anxiety that prompted support from the *New York Times* in its editorial praising police action in Sanger's Town Hall arrest. The same anxiety triggered a reappraisal after Sanger laid blame on the Catholic hierarchy. Catholics and Protestants shared the same support for the temperance and purity movements, when temperance was defined by individual moral restraint, but the Catholic Church was much less supportive when temperance was redefined as a mere ban on alcohol and saloons. The global Church did not view alcohol or any single vice as any more destructive than the weakness of moral character that caused the initial addiction.

In addition, the Catholic Church is based on a clear hierarchy that follows the monarchical model; the pope served above the bishops, who served above the priests, who led the people. The hierarchy of the Church was both celibate and male. Sanger was strongly opposed to all forms of religion, but she was especially opposed to the Catholic Church, which she believed was "oppressive" to women. While most Protestant leaders opposed Sanger's radicalism, they were sympathetic to Sanger's allusions to Catholic power and influence in American politics.

Since the 1880s, the number of Catholics in the United States increased dramatically relative to other Christian denominations, making it the largest single Christian church in the United States by 1912 with 12.6 million members. The largest Protestant denominations were Methodists (6.8 million), Baptists (5.6 million), United Lutherans (2.3 million), Presbyterians (1.9 million), Episcopalians (950,000), and the smaller denominations of Christian Reformed, United Brethren, Friends, Seventh-day Adventists, Jehovah's Witness, Pentecostals, and Latter-day Saints (1.5 million combined). Anti-Catholicism dated back from before the American Revolution, when Catholic churches were forbidden in all but a few colonies. It faded away but periodically returned during times of high immigration from traditionally Catholic nations. During the 1850s, the Know-Nothing Party was an anti-Catholic, anti-immigrant political party formed in reaction to the wave of Irish immigrants that came to the United States during the potato famine. The anti-Catholicism of the 1920s was in part due to the high number of Catholic immigrants from eastern and southern European countries. In part also, it was due to the postwar reaction against German authoritarianism, which some Protestants equated with the papal hierarchy.

Sanger successfully turned the issue of her arrest at the New York City Town Hall from one based on public decency and radicalism to one that pitted Catholics and Protestants against one another. Editors from both *The Outlook* and the *New Republic* came out with criticisms of police action in what they now referred to as the "Town Hall Raid." Specifically, they condemned the police for allowing themselves to be used as "puppets" of the Church and declared the entire event an unconstitutional violation of church-state relations. There was no evidence that the police had acted on any orders of the archbishop, but the public perception of collusion was enough to trigger some latent anti-Catholic hostilities that were already present.

THE SANGER EFFECT

Within months following her arrest at the New York City Town Hall, Sanger changed tactics in her effort to legalize contraceptives and contraceptive education. Rather than targeting capitalism or religion in general, Sanger focused her criticism directly at the Catholic Church. In her *Birth Control Review*, Sanger reflected on her arrest as an example of "the sinister control of the Roman Catholic Church, which attempts—and to a great extent succeeds—to control all questions of public and private morality in these United States." She further argued that the debate of contraceptives was actually a debate over religious and political freedom. In the same article, she claimed that "all who resent this sinister Church Control of life and conduct—this interference of the Roman Church in attempting to dictate the conduct and behavior of non-Catholics, must now choose between Church Control or Birth Control. You can no longer remain neutral. You must make a declaration of independence, or self-reliance, or submit to the dictatorship of the Roman Catholic hierarchy."

A contemporary historian, Kathleen Tobin, demonstrated in her book *American Religious Debate over Birth Control* that Catholics and Protestants were in strong agreement over the issue of contraception in 1921. Both groups were strongly supportive of the temperance and purity movements of the previous century, and both groups viewed contraceptives as destructive to the family and to standards of public morality. But after Sanger's Town Hall arrest and her subsequent charges of Catholic collusion with public officials, many mainline Protestant churches began to reevaluate their positions on the issue.

The first evidence of significant change in public perception came from John Sumner, secretary of the New York Society for the Suppression of Vice (which Anthony Comstock headed 30 years earlier). He repeated the traditional anti-Malthusian point that there was no evidence of overpopulation either in the United States or in Europe. He also maintained the traditional argument that the recent increase in the knowledge of birth control had led to changing attitudes to morality, weakening the marriage bond, which he linked to the increase in divorce rates. But then Sumner added, "We believe that where there is the probability of *diseased or mentally defective progeny*, or where the *health or life of the mother* would be endangered by child-bearing, *parents* should be advised against further issue and should be informed *personally by a licensed physician* of any known harmless means toward such a result." His point was that Sanger's radical defiance of the law was not necessary since women were already protected under the law, which already allowed doctors to prescribe contraceptives as needed. This last statement was significant because it marked formal recognition that birth control was no longer tied solely to morality and public decency. It was also a medical matter that could legally—and appropriately—be discussed between doctor and patient.

By 1924, Sanger was routinely addressing many large groups, including a meeting with 200 Yale Divinity School students, on the subject of birth control. She faced no further resistance from local authorities, and the question of whether birth control could be discussed in the public forum was decisively answered. During the same year, Sanger began receiving public support from ministers of less orthodox denominations, such as Unitarians and Universalists. She also received support from Reformed Jewish rabbis. Most of the mainline denominations retained their official opposition, but in 1925 and 1926 almost all of them created committees to look into the morality of contraception as medical innovation. The debate over birth control occurred not only in the secular public halls but also in the church halls.

The first official changes in denominational policies occurred in 1930. The Northern Baptist Conference allowed individual pastors to adapt to the constantly changing positions of medical innovation, meaning that each pastor could choose to endorse or not endorse birth control as one's parish indicated. Other denominations were much more explicit. The Universalists General Convention adopted a resolution that declared that the association of birth control with abortion and obscenity was based on broad misconceptions. Moreover, it urged members to repeal any provisions in the law that linked contraception to obscenity (including the Comstock provision) and encouraged individuals and churches to actively build birth control clinics under medical supervision to eradicate further public misconceptions on the issue. Within months, the American Unitarian Association, the New York East Conference of the Methodist Episcopal Church, and the Central Conference of American Rabbis all passed similar resolutions.

The final—and in some cases most significant—endorsement came from the Anglican Church Conference held in Lambeth, England. It is called by the archbishop of Canterbury once every 10 years and affects Anglicans all around the world. In August 1930, the conference passed a resolution explicitly permitting the use of contraceptives. This decision, later dubbed the **Lambeth Decision**, seemed to officially affirm the prediction made by Sanger eight years earlier that asserted that contraception was a major dividing point between Catholics and Protestants.

Sanger's prediction was only partially accurate. In 1931, the Presbyterian Conference rejected the use of contraception, citing its continuing view that contraception was a moral issue and that its increased presence in public debate resulted in higher divorce rates. The Missouri Synod Lutherans also condemned the use of contraception, and though the Southern Baptist Convention did not mention the topic explicitly, it pointedly condemned divorce as an increasing sin plaguing American society.

The Catholic Church also maintained its traditional position. At the end of 1930, Pope Pius XI promulgated the encyclical *Casti Connubii: On Christian Marriage*, which explicitly referred to contraception as a "sin against God." This followed an earlier statement from the Catholic magisterium in *Acta Apostolicae Sedis*, which argued that, "since therefore the conjugal act is destined primarily by nature for the begetting of children, those who in exercising it deliberately frustrate its natural effect and purpose, sin against nature and commit a deed which is shameful and intrinsically vicious."

Rather than strictly dividing Protestants and Catholics, the issue of contraception became the issue that distinguished between "liberal" and "orthodox" Protestant denominations. The northern Baptists separated from their southern counterparts on this issue. The Missouri Synod Lutherans separated from their German and United brethren, and Methodists separated from Presbyterians. For the next half century, individual congregational churches defined the rigor of their theology according to the position they took on contraceptive use.

AFTERMATH: BEFORE WORLD WAR II

Politically, Margaret Sanger was less successful in changing the legal environment for birth control. There were five congressional hearings on the subject of birth control legislation between 1931 and 1934, and Sanger spoke at all of them as the representative of the National Committee for Federal Legislation for Birth Control. The hearings resulted in the introduction of numerous bills sponsored by friendly congressmen, but none of them passed.

The Comstock Law remained unchanged, mostly because it dealt first with obscenity, contraception being only a minor provision. Sanger was effective in changing public sentiment on contraception to see it more as a medical issue than a moral issue, but she did little to change the public's overall sensitivity to obscenity and indecency. In some areas, such as movies, the pressure was to promote higher standards of decency. The

Hayes Production Code of 1930 set up strict guidelines of what could or could not be produced by Hollywood studios. It was not passed by Congress but was self-imposed as a preventive measure to ensure that the federal government would not step in. Public pressure for more decency in public media increased during the 1930s.

In practice, however, the public was obviously responding to birth control in some way—though it is unclear whether it was from natural or artificial methods. The birthrate from the 1930s fell below replacement level for the first time in American history, dropping from 2.13 percent in 1930 to 1.84 percent in 1933. By the middle of the decade, the Second Circuit Court of Appeals recognized the legality of doctors dispensing contraception with a prescription, even if the contraceptives and contraceptive information were shipped through the mail, in *United States v. One Package of Japanese Pessaries* (1936).

Dr. Hannah Stone, the director of one of Sanger's birth control clinics in New York City, ordered a package of rubber diaphragms from Japan, and they were confiscated en route by federal authorities under the Comstock Law. By this time, Sanger had developed a large support base, and her attorneys used this incident to overturn the Comstock Law. Sanger's lobbying efforts failed to secure legislative repeal, but a judicial reversal would have the same effect. The primary argument made by Sanger's attorneys was that birth control was necessary to protect women's health and well-being and that Dr. Stone's decision to prescribe diaphragms should not be covered by a law intended to protect against obscenity. Comstock's obscenity provision had no jurisdiction over medical decision making. The court agreed.

Sanger's attorneys failed to completely overturn Comstock, but they did succeed in carving out an explicit exception for physicians. Immediately after the *One Package* decision, Sanger lobbied the American Medical Association to change its Comstock-based position, which marginalized contraceptives. Within a year, the association formally recognized that a doctor's prescription of contraception was compatible with "proper medical practice." These efforts effectively established birth control as a legitimate and legal medical remedy.

In the years leading up to World War II, contraception had successfully entered into public debate as a medical issue. Federal law no longer regulated the distribution of contraceptive devices or materials through the mails, and the subject could be discussed and dispensed privately with impunity. Several state laws continued to explicitly prohibit contraception under their obscenity rules, but these laws were rarely enforced. Despite the legal laxity, a majority of churches still prohibited the use of artificial birth control as a personal sin, and Sanger could not completely remove contraception from questions of moral propriety.

At the same time, among academics especially, long traditions of eugenics and Malthusian arguments remained active influences in American policy. Eugenicists argued for more responsible matches but lobbied for sterilization of social dependents when possible. The neo-Malthusian arguments of overpopulation and resource scarcity became ever more popular as another world war loomed in the future. Both the extent of the war and the ideology of the prime enemy of the United States, Adolf Hitler, had significant impacts on the history of birth control from 1945 to the present.

CHAPTER 3

Birth Control Policy since 1945

The issue of birth control became a legitimate topic for public discussion during the 1930s, making its eventual legalization only a matter of time. The use and explanation of contraceptive methods by physicians was no longer legally marginalized and often received support from the academic and religious communities. Social scientists supported almost any technology that could improve the human condition, particularly if those technologies also promoted their eugenics and neo-Malthusian models of social engineering. Similarly, several mainstream Protestant and Reformed Jewish faith communities actively promoted birth control as an effective way to limit family size, avoid unnecessary economic hardships, free women of anxiety related to unwanted pregnancy, and generally take advantage of God's gift of science and technology to alleviate human suffering. The primary resistance to birth control continued to come mostly from the Catholic Church and the more orthodox Protestant denominations, both of which viewed contraceptives in moral rather than scientific terms. By the late 1930s, public sentiment was still divided on the issue, but the trend was moving toward more liberal access.

World War II had a major influence on legalizing contraceptive use both in the United States and abroad. Technological developments expanded the number of economic and other material resources available to researchers, helping to stimulate significant changes in the kinds and reliability of artificial birth control methods. In addition, the psychological impact of the war, its physical destructiveness, and plans for the future peace of the world all contributed greatly to the development of new **nongovernmental organizations** formed to promote the use of birth control around the world. Some of these organizations may have originally been formed with eugenics goals in mind, but by the 1960s they were motivated mostly by Malthusian-based models of overpopulation that influenced foreign policy, human rights, or environmental policy priorities.

By the time the baby-boomer generation reached the 1960s, oral contraceptives were legal and common in the United States, multinational organizations devoted millions of dollars dispensing them around the world, and federal policymakers debated how much money the federal government should spend on family planning services at home. A growing drug culture promoted a panoply of legal and illegal remedies for a variety of psychological and physical health issues. At the same time, public sensitivities to obscenity declined while the frequency of uncommitted sex outside of marriage increased in what was later referred to as the sexual revolution. The temperance and purity movements of the nineteenth century were all but forgotten, and a new sense of modern progress prevailed.

By 1968, contraception was no longer controversial. Instead, the new question for religious debate was whether induced abortions should be accepted as a modern medical innovation in the same way that contraception was. When the Vatican chose to research the issue of artificial birth control in 1965, many observers expected the Catholic Church to follow the example set by the majority of Protestant denominations and adapt a more science-centered position on reproductive technologies. Although few expected the pope to accept abortion, most assumed that birth control would be recognized as a modern practice. This was not the case. In 1968, the Catholic Church issued *Humanae Vitae*, which was an encyclical that not only rejected abortion as a grave sin but also reaffirmed contraception as a similar evil. The unpopular decision proved controversial.

By the 1980s, unlimited access to birth control and abortion was not only legal but also viewed as a civic right among many groups. Most state and federal health policies provided full funding for a variety of birth control methods with little successful political opposition. Dominant ethical questions were not based on obscenity or sexual morality but were instead limited to debates on the amounts of public funding, the protection of voluntary participation, and the prevention of health risks as they relate to consumer protection. Religious voices entering the debate were forced to frame their criticisms in those terms. Despite the demise of morality as a public safety issue, most criticism of contraceptive use and education remained deeply rooted to basic moral differences.

CONTRACEPTIVE RESEARCH AND DEVELOPMENT

During the 1920s, Margaret Sanger became a controversial voice for removing the moral stigmas associated with birth control and family planning. She was not, however, alone in this effort. As early as the 1910s, other less radical activists worked to decriminalize contraceptives. In 1915, Mary Ware Dennett formed the National Birth Control League, which was later disbanded to form the Voluntary Parenthood League. Dennett resisted Sanger's radical methods and argued instead that birth control be treated as a "purely scientific topic." She worked within the political system to challenge and change Comstock-based laws that prohibited publication of nonprurient sex education materials. For decades, Dennett and Sanger remained staunch rivals within the same movement for legal contraception.

Similarly, Dr. Robert Latou Dickinson, a longtime advocate for birth control, formed the Committee on Maternal Health in 1925. He feared the scandal associated with Sanger's activism and dedicated his time and finances to researching new methods of contraceptives in the name of medical research. With this approach, Dickinson attracted a great deal of money from philanthropists hoping to improve social welfare through scientific research. One such donor, Clarence Gamble, an heir to James Gamble (of Proctor and Gamble Corporation), provided Dickinson with large annual stipends, eventually leading to the research that produced the first oral contraceptive 30 years later.

Margaret Sanger also tried to flee from her more radical past by quitting all leadership positions in her American Birth Control League in order to concentrate on a new lobby group that she named the Clinical Research Bureau and the Committee of Federal Legislation in 1928. Like Dickinson, Sanger sought to capitalize on promoting birth control as a medical innovation rather than primarily as a tool of social reform. After the New York City Town Hall incident, her credibility as an advocate for scientific innovation increased, and she gained the support of John D. Rockefeller. Cooperation with Rockefeller marked a dramatic shift from radical to reformer for Sanger—just a decade earlier she wrote in *The Woman Rebel* that Rockefeller's assassination would help promote revolutionary change. By 1928, she was using wealthy industrialists to help fund her cause.

While the country was focused on foreign affairs during World War II, the National Birth Control League, the Committee on Maternal Health, and the Clinical Research Bureau finally merged together as a single conglomerate organization. Sanger and Dennett eventually joined forces under a new organization named the Birth Control Federation of America, which later was renamed the Planned Parenthood Federation of America in 1942. This group survives today as the largest single provider and lobbyist group for artificial contraceptives and abortion, with

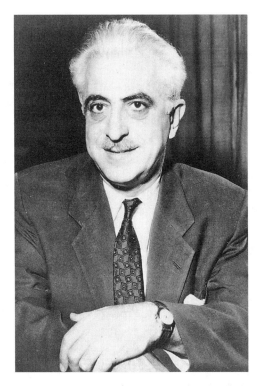

Gregory Pincus is remembered as one of the developers in the 1950s of the oral birth control pill, which contributed to the sexual revolution of the 1960s and the expansion of family planning all over the world. He cofounded the Worcester Foundation for Experimental Biology and was one of its directors for many years. (Library of Congress)

thousands of affiliate organizations, nearly 900 clinics nationwide, and a budget of over $1 billion.

After the war, Planned Parenthood added research funds to the money already provided for Dickinson's Committee on Maternal Health. The result was a new research team funded by the Committee on Human Reproduction, which was dedicated to the discovery of an anovulent oral contraception. For 10 years, scientists led by Gregory Pincus, John Rock, and Christopher Tietze worked on the project until they finally achieved a breakthrough in 1957. The resulting pill was approved for sale by the Food and Drug Administration (FDA) in 1960, forever changing the political environment of contraceptives and artificial birth control.

During the 1950s, birth control was no longer associated only with radical activists. With significant capital investment from large national organizations, contraception became a research industry. The invention of an oral contraceptive drug brought large pharmaceutical companies into the birth control lobby force. By the start of the 1960s, the new hurdle for birth control advocates was not legalization but rather government financing of contraceptives (and later of abortion) as part of a national social welfare policy.

POPULATION CONTROL AND FEDERAL POLICY

Prior to World War II, many arguments in favor of artificial birth control came from eugenicists who feared that the increase of "dependent" classes would eventually undermine the biological superiority of the "well-bred" classes—it was a future calamity that eugenicists often described as "**race suicide**." As late as 1939, Margaret Sanger maintained that "everything that advances the eugenic movement helps birth control as well." She complained that a pamphlet from the American Eugenics Society was not clear enough in its argument, explaining, "We know, without doubt, that certain groups should not reproduce themselves. Why not say so . . . we cannot improve the race until we first cut down production of its least desirable members. If we really believe this, let us say so plainly and bluntly."

Such explicit connection between advocates of eugenics and birth control was abruptly severed during World War II. In the 1930s, Nazi leader Adolf Hitler based his political support on the promise of creating a "master race" of pure Aryans. Relying heavily on the current research created by eugenics-based social scientists, Hitler's Third Reich launched many policies meant to alienate and segregate all non-Aryans but especially Jews. After the war began, German Nazi's implemented a plan to systematically murder these "dependent" groups. The resulting "Holocaust" left nearly 10 million Jews, Gypsies, and other non-Aryans dead. When the Nazi regime was finally defeated in 1945, the Western world was shocked by the discovery of hundreds of death camps of various sizes in German-occupied territories. From that point on, eugenics-based research was permanently associated with atrocity and dictatorship.

Malthusian based arguments of overpopulation were not tainted by events of World War II, and in some cases the conflict may have led to more support. The death of eugenics-based research created a vacuum that neo-Malthusians supporters could easily adapt to. For some social scientists, the war was an inevitable result of scarce natural resources in an overpopulated world. Likewise, the emerging Cold War reinforced the conviction that poverty and despair were the root cause of all extreme ideologies, such the Nazism and communism. In the late 1940s, the Soviet Union expanded its influence into nonindustrialized regions of the world in order to claim more resources. To the Malthusian-based social scientists, communist ideology was less important than the increasing problem of overpopulation, which made Third World nations more vulnerable to outside intrusion from Soviet-bloc nations.

This combination of new international tensions helped pushed birth control into the unexpected arena of American foreign policy. In 1952, John D. Rockefeller's grandson established the Rockefeller Population Council and appointed Frederic Osborn as its first president. Osborn had been a leader in the American Eugenics Society and had written *Preface to Eugenics* in 1940. After the war, he and Rockefeller recognized that eugenics was no longer marketable and concentrated instead on promoting birth control in African nations as a humanitarian effort to promote Western democracy.

There were other eugenics-to-population organizations that exploited the threat of a "population explosion" in African countries to garner support for their political objectives. The Rockefeller Population Council, however, tried to distance itself from the taint of political extremism and marketed itself instead in humanitarian terms. The global distribution of birth control was not merely a Cold War priority but should also be promoted as a solution to genuine human suffering. Regardless of Rockefeller's rhetoric, his humanitarian arguments remained closely tied to political goals.

The Population Council worked with the Rockefeller Foundation, the Ford Foundation, and International Planned Parenthood to lobby the World Health Organization and its member nations to solicit government funds for birth control in African countries. Since the issue was presented as a humanitarian need, other questions of moral decency were completely removed from discussion. In 1958, Sweden became the first Western nation to contribute government money ($366,000) toward family planning in a colonial state (in this case Ceylon). The trend for more government support was not far behind. In 1959, President Eisenhower appointed a special committee to study the effectiveness of the military aid program. Committee Chair General William Draper strongly recommended that the United States should spend more money on research on all human reproduction technologies, including birth control. Draper explained that "no realistic discussion" could ignore the fact that the economies of nonindustrialized nations were "being offset by increasingly rapid population growth."

FROM LEGALIZATION TO PUBLIC FUNDING

During his term in office, President Eisenhower did not directly support the recommendation of his commission. The president's hesitation was due mostly to a 1959 letter from the National Council of Catholic Bishops that opposed "any public assistant, whether at home or abroad to promote artificial birth control, abortion, or sterilization." After leaving office, though, Eisenhower's support for birth control became more explicit. In 1964, he joined former president Harry Truman to serve as cochair of the Planned Parenthood Federation. By that time, various lawmakers from both parties floated tentative proposals for using public funds to support birth control as a national health policy. The idea of a federal subsidy of domestic family planning programs was not immediately rejected.

Approval of oral contraceptives in 1960 by the FDA provided women with easy and discreet birth control, resulting in a 15 percent market share in the next five years. Despite the widespread use of artificial contraceptives, most states still had Comstock-like laws on the books limiting the distribution of contraception. Two states, Connecticut and Massachusetts, had laws that outlawed them altogether. These laws were not enforced—during the 80 years that the Connecticut law was on the books, only one case ever went to court. Nevertheless, the presence of any explicit prohibition posed a problem for future federal funding initiatives.

In *State v. Nelson* (1940), two Connecticut doctors and a nurse deliberately sought prosecution in order to challenge the constitutionality of the Connecticut law. The Second District Circuit Court of Appeals ruled that the Connecticut legislature was within its right to pass a law protecting public morals and ignored questions relating to the status of contraceptives as a medical or a moral matter. The court made reference to a similar test case in Massachusetts law and explicitly noted that both the Connecticut law and the Massachusetts law were constitutional because they reflected the power of states to "conserve the public safety and welfare, including health and morals" and such laws "may not be interfered with if [the State] has a real and substantial relation to those objects." Outside this single test case, no other unanticipated prosecution under the Connecticut Comstock-era law ever went forward.

By the 1930s, there was no real risk of prosecution under Comstock-era laws, but by the 1960s birth control advocates worked to remove all existing prohibitions in order to avoid possible obstacles for federal funding. Despite the lack of enforcement, lobbyists feared that some lawmakers might use the archaic laws to justify their refusal to spend state or federal money for reproductive services. As in 1940, their renewed effort to over-turn the old laws was initially problematic because the Supreme Court refused to hear theoretical challenges when there was no evidence that the state actually enforced the law. In order to overcome this technical hurdle, the executive director of Planned Parenthood of Connecticut, Estelle Griswold, arranged another test case by asking police to arrest her at one of her clinics. Attorneys for Planned Parenthood hoped that the 1960s Court would be more receptive to hearing the case if it were framed as a civil rights issue.

Planned Parenthood attorneys were correct. The Supreme Court agreed to hear the case and in *Griswold v. Connecticut* (1965) ruled in a seven-to-two decision that married persons had a constitutionally protected right to privacy and therefore could legally use contraceptives. The ruling proved extremely important later because no precedent for a "right to privacy" existed prior to *Griswold*, and it is not explicitly mentioned in the U.S. Constitution. Eight years later, in *Roe v. Wade* (1973), the Court expanded the right to privacy to include a woman's right to procure an abortion. Abortion, however, was not indicated in *Griswold*.

Although the general public experienced no immediate changes from the *Griswold* decision, lawmakers responded quickly. President Johnson's war on poverty focused on education, community action, and public health, and Planned Parenthood argued that federal funding for reproductive services should be on the forefront of urban poverty pro-grams. Johnson echoed this argument during his State of the Union Address in 1967, which served as a prelude for the "Foreign Assistant Act" dedicating $35 million to birth control programs overseas. Other amendments to the Social Security Act required all states to make contra-ceptives available through subsidies to family planning organizations (specifically Planned Parenthood). By 1968, the Office of Economic Opportunity spent $50 million to support 120 birth control clinics in the United States and $11 million to support clinics overseas.

With the federal government formally promoting family planning and subsidizing birth control inside and outside the country, few seemed to seriously question its moral suitability. Most observers were not surprised when Pope Paul VI agreed to a request by the Second Vatican Council to reconsider the morality of artificial birth control for the Catholic Church. Many onlookers, including many Catholics, expected the Church to change its views to better fit the practices of the modern scientific world. President Johnson's White House press secretary, Bill Moyers, remarked that "there is every evidence that even the Pope realizes the times are changing." This prediction, however, proved inaccurate. Even though federal agencies had begun to treat contraception purely in scientific terms, the Catholic Church (and a few other conservative Protestant denominations) continued to view the matter in strictly moral terms.

HUMANAE VITAE

The official teachings of the Catholic Church remained consistent on the issue of contraception throughout the rapid changes that occurred before and after World War II. By the 1960s, some prominent Catholics in the United States and in Europe pointed to the development of oral contraceptives as a medical breakthrough warranting a reappraisal by the Church. In his book *The Time Has Come*, Catholic gynecologist Dr. John Rock warned that "the population problem daily grows more destructive of the values to which all men aspire." He explained that neither the United States nor the United Nations was willing to spend the money necessary to effectively distribute birth control to Third World countries because both feared the power and influence of the Catholic Church. Dr. Rock had worked peripherally on the development of the progesterone-estrogen combination pill and believed that it provided a scientific way out of the old moral dilemma. He called on Catholic leaders to "extend the hand of fellowship toward those of other faiths" and work together to find an effective birth control solution acceptable by all.

Rock was not a priest or a theologian, but he was a respected physician and described himself as a devoted Catholic. His primary motivation was a fear of pending population explosion and ensuing poverty. Rock's argument for using modern contraceptives as a scientific solution was echoed by a minority of priests and bishops in the United States and Europe who, while not always calling for full tolerance of contraception, were nonetheless calling for an open discussion of the subject among the Church leaders. German Cardinal Julius Doepfner privately warned John XXIII that the "Church must change so that we do not impose on others sacrifices we know in our hearts are not necessary."

That year, in 1963, Pope John XXIII called a commission during the Second Vatican Council to study problems of the family, population, and birthrate. The group was formed in direct response to the growing pressures to address the "population explosion" of nonindustrialized countries in Africa and Asia. Pope John XXIII died shortly thereafter, but his successor, Pope Paul VI, continued the discussion with the qualification that he would make the final judgment on all recommendations.

After five years, the Papal Commission delivered a report to the Vatican. The majority opinion argued that modern medical science, combined with the changing status of women, necessitated tolerance of artificial methods of birth control to limiting rates of infant mortality and otherwise defer widespread poverty. There was also a minority report that reaffirmed the traditional Church interpretation that contraception was a grave sin. A month later, Pope Paul VI published the encyclical *Humanae Vitae* (On the Regulation of Birth), which rejected the majority view and instead reaffirmed the previous encyclical from 1930, *Casti Connubi*, condemning artificial contraception as a grave sin.

Catholics from Western nations were shocked by the decision, and a sizable proportion of academic theologians threatened to ignore the papal mandate. Within two months, the Canadian Conference of Catholic Bishops released the Winnipeg Statement, which said that individual Catholics should not be considered shut off from the Church if they were unable to accept the teaching of *Humane Vitae*. It further argued that individual Catholics could use contraceptives in good conscience provided that they first make an honest attempt to abide by the papal directives. The Winnipeg Statement contained no teaching authority and was not recognized by the Vatican, but it still reflected the strong immediate sense of dissent among Catholics in the West.

The central argument of *Humanae Vitae* is that marriage is an institution created by God and intended by God to serve as a vehicle for procreation. Sexuality has both unitive and procreative purposes and will increase the bond between husband and wife but only if it includes a mutual willingness to accept God's will in the transmission of life. Although the encyclical recognized that some families may want to limit the size of their families for a variety of legitimate reasons, including the physical and psychological health of the mother, it explicitly forbade artificial forms of birth control as intrinsically disordered to human nature.

The encyclical distinguished natural from artificial methods of birth control. Natural methods involve limiting the frequency of sexual intercourse during times when the woman is most likely to conceive. The Church tolerates natural family planning because it relies on individual restraint of both partners and therefore maintains moral discipline before God within the marriage. In addition, couples using natural methods of birth control always remained open to the "transmission of life" if God wills it.

The encyclical strongly condemned artificial methods of birth control because contraceptives separate the unitive from the procreative parts of the sexual act—without the openness to pregnancy, the marriage bond is removed from its future promise of a family, relegating sexual intercourse to a temporary act of sensual satisfaction alone. Pope Paul VI warned that artificial forms of contraception would trivialize sexuality and promote a "general lowering of moral standards," resulting in higher divorce rates, greater promiscuity, and a false sense of empowerment among women who might use sexuality as a tool. He also warned that sexuality for its own sensual sake will harm women because they will be seen by men as mere objects for sexual pleasure and not as necessary partners in the family. For these reasons, the encyclical also explicitly forbade without qualification abortion and sterilization.

Most observers lobbying for birth control had approached the issue from a medical perspective, and the moral arguments of *Humanae Vitae* initially appeared less relevant. Among Catholic leaders, however, the initial strong negative reaction was gradually replaced by broad consensus in later years. This trend became especially pronounced in the United States after the 1973 Supreme Court decision of *Roe v. Wade*, which forced all states to recognize abortion as another part of the legal right of privacy. A few notable Catholic theologians who had originally lobbied the Vatican to change its teaching later changed their views during the 1970s when statistics revealed doubled rates of divorce, premarital sex, and out-of-wedlock pregnancies. The Court decision to legalize abortion in all 50 states seemed to bear out the predictions warned by Paul VI. In 1976, the German Cardinal Doepfner wrote, "The more I think about it, the more I am convinced that the pope was right after all."

Although the Church hierarchy slowly grew more resolved in its support for *Humanae Vitae*, there was significant evidence to suggest that the Catholic laity remained hostile or indifferent to it. Estimates of Catholic women using oral contraceptives during the 1970s ranged from 40 to 80 percent. More significantly, the unchanging opposition amid widespread practice cost Catholic leaders part of their voice in public debates. Advocates for birth control and abortion rights pointed to *Humanae Vitae* as evidence that the Catholic Church was out of touch with modern science, hostile to modern change, and apathetic to the rights of modern women. American presidents and policymakers no longer waited on the Church to change its position before incorporating family planning measures into their federal budgets.

Although the actual number of practicing Catholics increased during the 1970s and 1980s, there were fewer public figures championing the mandates of the Church as it related to artificial birth control. The political influence of American bishops became fragmented and weaker. As birth control became more deeply identified with scientific innovation, woman's health, and global poverty, the moral perspective provided by conservative critics became increasingly less influential with American policymakers.

ABORTION VERSUS BIRTH CONTROL

After 1968, contraceptives were not only legal but also effectively isolated from moral arguments. On the international level, family planning services were marketed as humanitarian weapons in the fight against overpopulation and resource depletion. They became inextricably linked with foreign policy as the United States endeavored to stabilize those nonindustrialized nations who were most susceptible to communist insurrections. On the domestic front, birth control was tied to maternal health and was promoted as one of many tools to fight the problems of urban poverty. These forces ensured broad acceptance of contraceptives among policymakers, but they did not ensure any special priority over other social welfare tools. Advocates worked to change that in the 1970s.

Legalized abortion changed the national debate dramatically. Following the path used to legalize contraception, family planning groups began pushing abortion as the new legal front for medical innovation. Back in 1959, the American Law Institute proposed a model criminal code for states to reform their existing laws against abortion. At the time, such proposals found little traction. The situation changed, however, as soon as birth control began being debated within the Catholic Church. By June 1967, the American Medical Association reversed its former opposition to abortion and declared that abortions could be a legitimate medical procedure in certain circumstances.

Between 1967 and 1970, 13 states modified their laws to allow abortion in cases where the woman's life was at risk or for cases of rape, incest, and severe defect. Between 1970 and 1972, four more states lifted the ban altogether, allowing women to procure an abortion at will. The tide began to shift, though, after Catholic bishops and laypeople led a large-scale campaign to repeal these laws, involving numerous organizations including the National Right to Life Committee. In 1972, the New York state legislature voted to overturn its recent legalization but was vetoed by Governor Nelson Rockefeller. Attempts in Michigan and North Dakota to repeal their abortion laws were met with strong voter rejection of three-to-one and four-to-one margins.

Birth control lobbyists responded with their own political campaigns. Planned Parenthood joined women's rights groups to oppose the Catholic-led opposition to legalize abortion at the national level. They argued that the Catholic Church and other foes of abortion reflected institutional sexism by denying women the freedom to pursue their own ambitions without the shackles of pregnancy and childbirth. The argument helped tie both contraception and abortion together as an essential right of women, necessary to free them from the economic and moral dependence on men.

For many observers, this brand of feminism echoed the same radical language used by Margaret Sanger during the 1910s. Decades earlier, birth control advocates made a deliberate effort to escape the taint associated by Sanger's early activism and instead worked diligently to transform the issue of birth control into the morally neutral context of medical and humanitarian innovation. By the late 1960s, though, a younger generation of advocates seemed to welcome the return to more radical tones.

The difference between the two eras was mostly a matter of global context. Whereas the 1920s was dominated by general opposition to radicalism following World War I and the Russian Revolution, the 1960s was dominated by a broad public support for civil rights movements that emerged during the 1950s to target racial injustice in the South. Landmark legislative successes in 1964 and 1965 (the Civil Rights Act and the Voters Rights Act, respectively) led race-based rights activists to broaden their attention to other examples of injustice. Women's rights groups emerged in the wake of the racial rights agenda and easily assumed the same language as a coequal civil rights movement.

The general public of the 1960s was not necessarily sympathetic with the new radical language. But certain sectors (especially among academics, lawyers, and judges) were much more sensitive to civil rights in its broad context. Antiabortion groups were gaining ground in 1972, but the Supreme Court reversed their efforts in 1973 in *Roe v. Wade*, where the Court ruled that the "right to privacy" guaranteeing women the right to contraceptives also guaranteed them the right to procure an abortion. This was a major victory both for advocates of birth control and for women's rights.

There were two major effects of combining abortion and contraception as equivalent rights. First, opponents of abortion were forced to choose their priorities. Most Protestant denominations viewed birth control as a medical innovation but held abortion as the willful destruction of human life. When placed in tandem with each other, many denominations chose to be even more supportive of birth control as a necessary alternative to abortion. The Catholic hierarchy remained explicitly opposed to both contraceptives and abortion, but of the two, they also deemed abortion as the more pressing concern. In deference to the Catholic-Protestant coalition that emerged to combat proabortion forces, the Catholic Church remained mostly silent on the issue of contraception during the 1970s and 1980s.

The second significance was that the Court's "right to privacy" guaranteed a constant legal link between contraception and abortion. After 1973, not only was birth control a humanitarian weapon in the war against overpopulation and urban poverty, but it had also become an essential legal right guaranteeing women's equality. Lawmakers who may have been hesitant to spend state and federal dollars on social welfare projects were suddenly more conscious of the political consequences of withholding birth control resources for fear of violating women's civil rights. After the 1970s, lawmakers from both parties maintained relatively consistent state and federal budgetary support for birth control services, even when they fought openly over funding for abortion services.

FUNDING AND CULTURE WARS

In 1970, President Richard Nixon signed Title X of the Public Health Service Act, creating Public Law 91-572, "Population Research and Voluntary Family Planning Programs." The federal program is entirely dedicated to providing education and access to birth control and other family planning services. The law guaranteed special priority for women in low-income families. The program falls under the Office of Public Health and Science, which is under the Office of Family Planning. After 40 years, the funding has increased annually to support a network of more than 4,500 clinics within state and local health departments with an outreach of 5 million women.

Since *Roe v. Wade*, birth control has taken a backseat to abortion as the frontline issue in debates between regulation of public morality versus government funding and support of women's health care. As a political issue, birth control remains in a separate category from abortion in terms of public funding for family services. In 1984, Republican President Ronald Reagan announced the "Mexico City Policy," which forbade the use of foreign aid money sent for family planning services to be used for abortion services. The policy was maintained when the elder President Bush took office in 1989 but was immediately reversed under Democratic President Bill Clinton in 1993. When the younger President Bush was elected in 2000, he quickly reinstated the Mexico City policy, which stayed in effect throughout his administration. In 2009, one of President Barack Obama's first acts was to again reverse the policy. Foreign assistance for other artificial birth control methods remained untouched throughout all five administrations.

The distinction extended both outside and inside the United States. Since the Hyde Amendment in 1977, Congress has explicitly prohibited the direct use of Title X funds to pay for abortion services. In 1987, President Reagan took an additional step by issuing an executive order forbidding federal counselors and health workers at Title X–funded clinics from referring clients to abortion providers. Dubbed the "gag rule" by abortion lobbyists, Democrats vowed to overturn the order when they retook the White House. Like the Mexico City policy, each subsequent president has either affirmed or overturned the "referral" policy, depending on his party—Republicans supporting the prohibition of referrals and Democrats opposing it. Yet throughout the nine administrations since President Johnson, Title X and related state funding for birth control as a public health policy promoting family planning initiatives has either increased or remained the same.

Recent innovations in contraceptive technology led to questions about whether certain birth control methods actually worked as abortifacients. The question of whether a contraceptive avoids pregnancy or terminates a pregnancy at the very earliest stages has serious religious implications. During the 1990s, several conservative Protestant denominations reconsidered their support for birth control over the prospect that they may be linked to abortion. These concerns were magnified after the FDA approved certain "emergency contraceptives" that women could take after sexual intercourse. Several pro-life physician groups with members of all faiths, including Physicians for Life, publicly refused to prescribe or administer contraceptives that could act as abortifacients.

In recent years, since the 2000s, most political debate has focused on whether federal agencies should force insurance agencies and pharmacies to include all forms of contraceptives in their coverage, including emergency contraceptives. Other debates have arisen over whether the federal government should force all doctors and pharmacists to provide any contraceptive on patient request. Both debates deal with questions that pit physicians' freedom of conscience or religious convictions against women's right to access medical devices affecting their reproductive options. Both debates remain divided largely along partisan lines. When the line between birth control and abortion becomes blurred, the resulting debate generally focuses less on medical matters and more on political and religious convictions.

Social acceptance of birth control is no longer a public debate, but larger moral questions that weigh public health and civil rights against public morality remain undecided. The next section considers recent debates over the past two decades that relate directly to questions of consumer protection and women's health, public funding domestically and as a matter of foreign policy, legal questions of voluntariness, informed consent, and gender differences and inequities relating to male and female contraceptive options.

Contemporary Controversies and Issues Relating to Birth Control

CHAPTER 4

Consumer Protection

The question of safety has followed chemical-based contraceptives since their inception. In the United States, an anonymous birth control manual from 1855 warned that contraceptive "drugs and chemicals" cause side effects ranging from inflammation of the reproductive and urinary organs to inexcusably bad breath. The author concluded that these side effects "render their use repugnant to the feelings and moral sensibilities of all virtuous and honorable people" and recommended, instead, a nonchemical alternative.

The fear of harmful side effects almost always accompanies moral criticisms of birth control. After describing the spiritual damage that birth control inflicts on home and family, opponents like Anthony Comstock almost always included examples of the dangerous side effects of both chemical and mechanical forms of contraceptives. Within a few generations, though, that tactic backfired. Margaret Sanger took advantage of the generalized concerns for women's health and shifted the nature of the debate with the warning that health risks associated with pregnancy were far greater than the side effects of contraceptives. Society was harmed by the lack of safe birth control, and women's health was better protected when they had professional advice on proper birth control methods. Yet in the early 1910s, even Sanger warned against the reckless use of chemical-based methods and recommended only mechanical solutions.

After World War II, medical technologies improved significantly, and both doctors and the public alike placed greater faith in the utility of pills and other chemical solutions for everyday ailments. Birth control advocates like Alan Guttmacher hailed oral contraceptives as an "important part of medical care" equal to other breakthroughs, such as penicillin or aspirin, perhaps even more important because birth control fulfilled a basic social need that had previously been ignored. He added that there was "no evidence that [birth control] causes cancer or any other disease."

Guttmacher's optimism may have been a little premature in hindsight, and there was a small segment of the population who still feared unexpected side effects of using chemicals to stop pregnancy. Those were the people whom Guttmacher most wanted to reach. He launched numerous publicity campaigns to provide women with scientific justification for the strong public demand for the easy, discreet method of oral contraceptives. This enthusiasm for a safe modern solution to an age-old problem naturally pushed latent concerns about public safety to the background.

By the start of the 1970s, most women had used one or more chemical contraceptive methods at some point in their lives, regardless of the apparent risks. Over time, however, the sheer number of consumers ensured that harmful side effects would eventually be noticed. By the early 1990s, after the generation of women who had used birth control throughout most of their adult lives started reaching the age of menopause, several negative health trends began to emerge—some quite serious. Predictably, consumer protection groups filed a series of lawsuits targeting pharmaceutical companies that produced contraceptives.

Unlike the opponents of Anthony Comstock's time, the lawsuits of the 1990s were not filed to prohibit legal access to birth control. The courts had already affirmed legality, and public consensus accepted birth control as a normal part of health care. Instead, the primary motivation for the lawsuits was to force drug makers to prove that their commitment to consumer safety outweighed the drug's market value. A flurry of lawsuits resurrected old questions about the safety of contraceptives—but as a consumer protection issue and not as a matter of public morality. This morally neutral approach received broad consideration from people of all ideological perspectives.

ORIGINAL PROMISE FOR WOMEN'S HEALTH

Birth control was legalized largely on the promise that it would provide greater protection for women's health. Once it moved away from the realm of decency and public morality and was framed instead as a public welfare issue, the general public provided ample support. Margaret Sanger argued that fewer babies meant that a greater percentage of those born would be better cared for, unhealthy women would be less likely to suffer complications from uncontrolled pregnancies, poor women would not be forced to divide inadequate provisions among as many mouths, and young women would be able to establish healthier homes before bringing new children into them. More important, families with hereditary defects could protect future generations by preventing those genetic traits from being passed on.

In addition to Sanger's approach, another strain of the public safety argument believed that the demand for birth control almost always outweighed women's fears of health risks. Women have looked for ways to control their reproduction cycles for thousands of years, and that natural demand would not be weakened by legal restrictions or religious opposition. Depriving women of safe and legal methods of birth control only pushed them to pursue underground markets, forcing women to resort to unsafe methods offered by unscrupulous and unregulated vendors. By contrast, broad legal access to medically guaranteed birth control options safeguarded public health in general and women's health in particular. Both strains of the public safety argument were used to justify continual government support for family planning services since the late 1960s.

Regardless of the rhetorical confidence, the truth remains that there are always side effects from birth control. From the start, the public expected to face some risk with new oral contraceptives, but the first indications of serious health risks came not from chemical-based contraceptives but instead from a mechanical intrauterine device (IUD). In 1974, the Food and Drug Administration (FDA) suspended support for the Dalkon Shield brand of IUD after more than 100 women suffered spontaneous abortions, seven of whom later died from related complications. Advocates for legal and government-funded contraceptives had devoted considerable energy promoting artificial birth control as a solution to public health problems, so the news of mortally harmful side effects created a national sensation. The product was pulled from the market, and a class-action law suit was filed. The manufacturers of Dalkon Shield improved the IUD design, marketed it successfully three years later with few noticeable side effects. Nevertheless, the memory of the initial Dalkon Shield caused many women in the United States to steer away from using IUDs for almost a decade. This had an unexpected consequence of encouraging even more women to rely exclusively on chemical-based methods.

UNKNOWN VARIABLES

One difficulty facing pharmaceutical companies is the predominance of unknown variables. For example, even in the twenty-first century, scientists do not know exactly how mechanical IUDs work. Researchers cannot determine if it is the shape of the IUD or the chemical makeup of the materials that prevents the conception. Similarly, scientists are also unclear exactly how the progesterone-only family of contraceptives works—research has not definitively proven whether the chemical prohibits conception or whether it prohibits implantation of the ovum (which could destroy the ovum after fertilization). Since the process of conception always occurs with living human subjects, it is very difficult to test these questions with absolute certainty.

The relatively recent discovery of oral contraceptives means that scientists have little evidence to measure the impact of long-term use on women's health. Only a few studies have questioned the impact of early contraceptive use on women's later ability to conceive. Since conception can often be difficult to achieve in the best of circumstances, researchers cannot easily isolate the variables in a typical woman's life to know whether her inability to conceive is a result of long-term use of contraceptives or due to some other unidentified environmental factor. Smoking, drinking, and other legal or illegal drugs may contribute significantly to fertility, but the degree to which the sustained use of artificial contraceptives mitigates or magnifies those factors remains unclear. Since the actual process of chemical or mechanical contraception (such as IUDs) is not absolutely known, then there are too many unknown variables to be able to establish with certitude any long-term effects of continued use on other systems in the body.

BIRTH CONTROL AND CANCER RISK

The American Cancer Society reports that cancer rates among all populations increased steadily between 1975 and 1989. Yet after 1999, those rates have generally decreased. One major exception to these trends is in the rates of breast and cervical cancers in women. After a period of no significant change prior to 1980, the incidents of breast cancer rose steadily between 1980 and 1987 and then, contrary to prevailing trends, rose again from 1999 to 2006. The dates of increase correspond to similar trends of increased access to oral contraceptives among women a generation earlier. While no direct evidence can link cancer to birth control, the correlations suggest that women who used oral contraceptives for 10 years or more were more likely to develop breast cancer in their late 30s. Additionally, women who had not used contraceptives for a period of 10 years or more had the same cancer rates as the general population. These correlations indicate that the habitual use of oral contraceptives increased the risks.

Researchers suspect that some cancer cells rely on the fast growth rates of sex hormones to develop and multiply. Most oral contraceptives use a synthetic form of progesterone to trick the body into thinking it is already pregnant, thereby delaying (sometimes indefinitely) additional release of ovum. Successful contraception requires a constant presence of progesterone to prevent fertilization, increasing the likelihood of developing sex hormone–dependent cancers. Whereas the general population is exposed to progesterone for short terms of nine months, women taking oral contraceptives may expose themselves to the hormone continuously for periods of years at a time or even decades.

A 1996 study concluded that oral contraceptives increase the cancer risks for all women but especially for those who began use as teenagers and for women with family histories of cancer. Another study in 2003 affirmed this positive correlation and further suggested that cancer rates were highest among young women who had used oral contraceptives within five years of the diagnosis. These and other studies, however, are correlational in nature. Research into the direct causal connections between progesterone and cancer is extremely difficult to administer since the test subjects involve living humans.

INCOMPLETE DISCLOSURE

Cancer is one of the most researched medical ailments in American science, and it is not surprising that researchers would uncover some carcinogenic risks in oral contraceptives. Other long-term risks, however, are less well known. The rates of long-term sterility, mood disorders, or other ailments remain largely unexamined. Critics argued that the advocates of birth control focus so much attention on the sociopolitical advantages of birth control that they unwittingly and uncritically encouraged acceptance of a potentially dangerous drug.

The risks associated with oral contraceptives are not publicized as thoroughly as the potential benefits of controlled reproduction, but history has shown that birth control is not simply matter of medical health. Sanger and other feminists argued that contraceptives are necessary for women to be able to control their lifelong vocations—access to birth control is a fundamental civil right, and unexpected or unintended motherhood undermines women's rights and freedom. For these groups, the pressure to promote the benefits of birth control strongly outweighs other incentives to fully disclose potential side effects of long-term (or widespread public) use. Most family planning organizations devote most of their resources to educating the public on the necessity of birth control, leaving the discussion of potential side effects as an unavoidable encumbrance.

Similarly, the manufacturers of oral contraceptives have few incentives to research the potential side effects of long-term use. The market share of

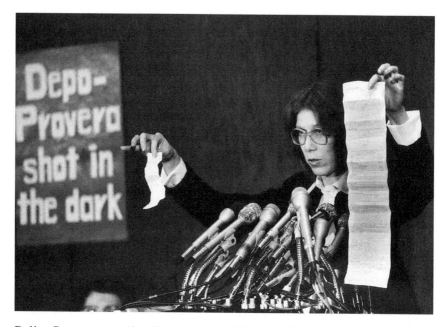

Belita Cowan, executive director of the National Women's Health Network, holds a Washington news conference to announce her organization will bring a lawsuit against the maker of the birth control injection called Depo-Provera for those who have been injured by its use. Cowan is holding instructions that have to do with the use of the drug; the one in her right hand is packed with the drug, and in her left hand is the one that the doctors receive. (AP Photo/ Ira Schwarz)

birth control products is in the billions of dollars. Their products reach a broad demographic (all women in their childbearing years, whether they are healthy or not), and the competition between companies to dominate that consumer base can be fierce. The FDA requires testing for short-term side effects, but long-term effects require many years to research, and the results may not be conclusive. Drug companies have little reason to publish inconclusive research that might inadvertently taint a product. The tainted brand of Dalkon Shield serves as a great disincentive to fund or fully disclose research into long-term health risks of contraceptives.

In addition, state and federal governments have little power to regulate contraceptives on the probability of future health risks alone. The FDA requires clinical tests for new drug patents, and manufacturers are required to report adverse drug reactions quarterly (or within two weeks if the reaction leads to death), but these safeguards are useful only for short-term reactions. The number of unknown variables in an individual's lifestyle makes long-term reactions very difficult to detect. The FDA is ill equipped to protect consumer from possible carcinogens.

As a result of these corporate and regulatory obstacles, the most common tool of consumer protection is the class-action lawsuit. If enough victims of an unsafe product join together to file a claim against a drug company, then the legal system could potentially levy a substantial financial penalty. The fear of such lawsuits does provide drug companies with an incentive to thoroughly investigate and disclose potential long-term risks. Unfortunately, the same fear of future litigation may also encourage drug companies to avoid long-term research because the results are almost always inconclusive. A report containing false negatives might prevent a company from releasing a new drug that might actually be quite safe. Or, worse, future litigants who suffered reactions from unknown variables unrelated to their drug might still use the inconclusive research to support their claim against the drug company.

During the late 1980s and early 1990s, tobacco companies were sued by various states that argued that the companies knew about the harmful effects of smoking yet refused to disclose the information. The tobacco companies argued that in strict scientific terms, the causal connection between smoking and lung cancer could not be absolutely established and thus that they should not be held liable for any legal claims. Yet the prevalence of strong correlational data combined with the inclusive research data was sufficient to place the tobacco companies in a losing position. Since then, pharmaceutical companies have also been hesitant to conduct research for results that are not absolutely essential.

TARGET MARKETS

In addition to incomplete disclosure, critics also argue that pharmaceutical companies inappropriately market their contraceptives to expand their consumer demographic. The 1936 case of *One Package* argued that contraceptives were appropriately discussed in the privacy of a doctor's office. In the 1960s, Alan Guttmacher and others argued that oral contraceptives provide women with a discreet way of practicing birth control without letting anyone but the married woman and her doctor know about it. By the 2000s, however, birth control was being advertised in teen fashion magazines, during prime-time television spots, and on public billboards. The target audience for birth control is now younger, and the collateral benefits of extended use have expanded to include more regular menstruation, acne prevention, and increased concentration. While the potentially harmful long-term side effects are often ignored because of inconclusive results, the breadths of subsidiary positive side effects are heavily marketed without similar hesitation.

A 2007 study of eight marketing websites maintained by major manufacturers of oral contraceptives revealed that most brands claimed that their products were 99 percent effective when used properly. In addition, though, the most common motivational cues focused on their brand's enhancement of a young woman's freedom, personal control, intelligence, and physical attractiveness. The Yaz/Yasmin brands specifically targeted teens by including antiacne ingredients with the progesterone to produce a product that prevents pregnancy and reduces pimples.

Critics argue the teen demographic is not adequately informed to be able to engage in an educated risk assessment before choosing whether to use a particular oral contraceptive. Direct-to-consumer marketing practices potentially sidestep the professional advice of a physician and take advantage of teen girls who may already be vulnerable to self-esteem issues and may unfairly promote consumption of a product that could result in long-term health risks.

Some unexpected critics have arisen from women's rights organizations and argue that the emphasis on oral contraceptives has unfairly focused on women and ignored the responsibility of men. Since the outbreak of the AIDS epidemic in the 1980s, condom use has been most associated with protection against sexually transmitted diseases and not primarily as a birth control method. The result is that the responsibility of birth control has fallen exclusively on young women, who generally rely on chemical methods and who may or may not be fully educated on the associated health risks. Some woman rights advocates have begun to challenge drug companies to devote more resources into an oral contraceptive for men that would render their sperm infertile. But the existing demand for oral contraceptives among women remains very high, while the demand for male alternatives among men remains low. Pharmaceutical companies have few incentives to alter their long-term business plans.

CONCLUDING THOUGHTS

For decades, the primary question for birth control policy was whether their broad access would undermine the moral health of society. Critics of the past challenged the harmful moral effects of sexual activity outside the institution of marriage and viewed birth control as an assault on decency. Those arguments lose potency when the issue is redirected to questions of medical science and physical health. The morally neutral context of modern debates ignores the advisability of sexuality between high school–aged teens and focuses primarily on physical safety and emotional maturing to gauge whether teens are educated enough to make medical decisions that could potentially affect their long-term health.

The new debates remain equally charged because the underlying motivations may not be as far removed from the past as it appears. The old arguments did not die, and the religious-based criticisms did not fade. Instead, they are often rearticulated into more socially acceptable terms of full disclosure and consumer safety. Former questions of moral health frequently guide a broad range of questions challenging the role of birth control in relation to women's health and consumer protection.

CHAPTER 5

Government Policy

Birth control is legal in the United States. This is true whether the method is artificial, natural, mechanical based, or chemical based. The Supreme Court's decision in *Griswold v. Connecticut* (1965) stipulated that no state could deny married women the right to practice birth control in the privacy of their own homes. This right was reaffirmed by *Eisenstadt v. Baird* (1972), which guaranteed access to contraceptives to all women—married or unmarried. Some years later, the Court further extended the right in *Lawrence v. Texas* (2003) when it ruled that no state has a legitimate reason to intrude on the personal and private lives of individuals, particularly as it relates to sexual conduct in "the most private of places, the home." For more than 40 years, there have been no serious challenges to *Griswold* or the legal construct on which it is based. Similarly, the right to practice birth control remains untouched by political activism or public pressures. There is no effort to ban the manufacture, sale, or distribution of birth control devices, literature, or access to clinics.

Yet the question of legality is complicated by its companion issue of government funding. Legalizing access is not the same as guaranteeing access: "legalizing" birth control means that women who have the resources may use contraceptives at will, and "guaranteeing access" means that the government will provide contraceptive services for people who are unable to afford it. Guarantees involve a financial commitment, which complicates public support. It is one thing to tolerate (legalize) a practice that is contrary to your faith, but it is a different matter to ask those who oppose the practice on moral ground to pay for it through taxes. When federal or state agencies choose to guarantee women full and complete access to birth control, then taxpayers are forced to pay for its distribution. The issue of civil rights becomes a more complicated question of voluntariness once public money is involved in the equation.

GOVERNMENT FUNDING AND OBJECTIVITY

The connection between legalization and public funding was formed at the very beginning of legalization. The plaintiffs in *Griswold* deliberately courted arrest in order to provide the courts an opportunity to strike down all remaining Comstock-era laws. Connecticut had not prosecuted birth control clinics for more than half a century, nor were the Comstock laws of other states being enforced. The motivation for seeking arrest was to forcibly remove all remaining legal prohibitions so that lobbyists could actively seek funding for family planning resources in government-subsidized clinics. As long as the laws prohibiting birth control remained on the books, lawmakers were free to use the prohibitions as an excuse to deny funding for contraceptive services at government-sponsored clinics.

The goal of the *Griswold* plaintiffs was not to legalize but to subsidize. In 1965, the same year that the Supreme Court published its decision, advocates for Planned Parenthood had already begun petitioning President Johnson to include funding for contraceptives to low-income households as part of his "war of poverty." Within two years, Johnson signed the Social Security Amendments of 1967, which stipulated that at least 6 percent of maternal and child health care funds be spent on family planning services. By 1970, President Nixon signed the Public Health Service Act, in which Title X provided funding for "population research and voluntary family planning programs." Since then, the federal government has continually subsidized contraceptives and other related family planning services for more than 4,500 clinics, reaching more than 75 percent of local counties nationwide. Recent funding for Title X has exceeded $300 million and typically grows 3 to 5 percent per year.

In addition to Title X, most states also have equivalent programs with a wide range of funding amounts. The total expenditures for government-funded family planning programs in 2006 was $1.85 billion. More than 70 percent of those funded came from joint programs between the federal government and state agencies. For example, California's Family PACT Program provides free contraceptives to women with annual incomes up to 200 percent of the national poverty level and has a budget of over $430 million a year, much of which comes from federal sources. By contrast, New York's family planning programs share a budget of around $40 million a year, but it is spread throughout a larger $1.1 billion health care program.

Where does this money go? Nationally, 9 million women received publicly funded contraceptive services in 2010. California alone serves more than 2.5 million women in a variety of health care venues operating as community clinics, on college campuses, in hospitals, and in Planned Parenthood clinics. By far, the single largest recipient of both state and federal funds is Planned Parenthood of America, which received approximately 80 percent of the business provided by federally funded clients. The national networks owes more than a third of its $1.18 billion budget to Title X subsidies and a somewhat lesser amount to state agencies.

Some critics contend that the amount of government money devoted to family planning creates a conflict of interest among practitioners and policymakers. The leading source of information that lawmakers use to evaluate the impact of contraceptives on public health comes from the same groups that receive government money. Planned Parenthood and the Guttmacher Institute are leading sources for family planning information, yet they are also the largest recipients of government funds. Critics who oppose contraception on moral grounds are naturally quick to point out these conflicts, while supporters of Planned Parenthood and the Guttmacher Institute often dismiss such criticism as prejudiced rhetoric.

"CIVIL RIGHTS" OR "PUBLIC HEALTH"

Early advocates for the legalization of artificial birth control argued that it was a woman's right to freely choose whether to become pregnant. In terms of government funding, however, the primary argument focuses on the impact of unintended pregnancies on public health. The Guttmacher Institute advertises that each dollar spent on contraception for low-income households saves four dollars in other government subsidized health programs, such as Medicare. The argument rests on the assumption that the family planning programs reduce the number of low-income children, thereby lowering the financial burden of taking care of those children as they grow and mature.

Although family planning lobbyists for government subsidies rest their pleas on the needs of public health, the linkage between birth control and women's rights remains a constant pressure on lawmakers. Failure to provide money for family planning can be argued as a failure to protect the special needs of women. Early activists, such as Margaret Sanger, routinely warned that unwanted pregnancies obstruct a woman's ability to fully participate in education and the economy without the burden of parental responsibilities. Planned Parenthood describes itself as "pro-woman" because it advocates for legalization and funding of both birth control and abortion services at state and federal levels.

The result of this tacit association between birth control and women's rights is that government subsidies of birth control remained steady. Most government-run family planning agencies are protected from significant budget cuts because politicians are hesitant to appear insensitive to either women's rights or public health care costs. There is, nevertheless, some pressure from groups who oppose government subsidies on moral or religious grounds. Mostly, the opposition arises when birth control is linked with abortion. For example, Planned Parenthood receives about 10 percent of its revenue from performing abortions. Abortion opponents who might otherwise support contraceptives may still lobby their representatives to defund birth control because they fear that the money could indirectly be used to support abortions.

An effort to separate public money used for birth control from money used for abortion services began almost immediately after abortion became legalized. The Supreme Court decision of *Roe v. Wade* (1973) opened the door for federal funding of abortion, just as *Griswold* had paved the way for federal funding of birth control. In 1976, Illinois Congressman Henry Hyde added an amendment to a federal health care bill prohibiting any funds from being used to pay for abortions. The addendum passed the House by a sizable majority, and similar amendments have been added to each new federal health care bill ever since. The rider is now dubbed the Hyde Amendment and has become a standard item for all health care bills where money could potentially be used to subsidize family planning services. There is a tacit agreement between both parties to include this provision each funding cycle.

In the 1980s, President Reagan announced while in Mexico City that he had issued an executive order prohibiting the use of any foreign moneys designated for birth control to be also used for abortion services. Dubbed the Mexico City policy, Reagan expanded the Hyde Amendment to apply to overseas aid. Unlike the Hyde Amendment, however, the Mexico City policy had little public presence since most Americans rarely saw how foreign aid is actually spent overseas. The result is that the issue became strongly politicized as a pro-life versus pro-choice litmus test.

Since the 1980s, the Republican Party has aligned itself with a pro-life agenda that opposes abortion on principle and seeks to limit the conditions in which abortions could be legally performed. By contrast, the Democratic Party has aligned itself with a pro-choice agenda that supports abortion and seeks to provide easy access to abortion on demand with no restrictions.

Since 1988, each Republican president has reaffirmed Reagan's Mexico City policy and prohibited the use of foreign aid for abortion services. Similarly, since 1992, each Democratic president has overturned Reagan's policy and has permitted unrestricted use of family planning aid to be used for both birth control and abortion services. The net effect of these political conflicts is that any discussion of abortion in relation to subsidies for birth control almost always guarantees a highly charged debate.

Public support for birth control subsidies does not carry over to abortion. Abortion advocates, such as Planned Parenthood and the Guttmacher Institute, oppose provisions that might limit access to abortion because they hold the freedom to choose an abortion as a basic woman's right. That association between "abortion" and "rights" is so strong that is becomes a political liability within discussions of public funding of birth control. It is one of the reasons why birth control advocates take care to justify continued government subsidies in terms of public health only. The unintended consequence of explicitly linking birth control to civil rights often raises unwanted associations with abortion and could kill the pending legislation. As such, public funding for birth control is usually described as a "cost-savings" measure intended to protect the public health by preventing unwanted pregnancies.

"Family Planning" or Eugenics

In the United States, birth control and abortion are associated with individual freedom and a woman's "right to choose." Voluntary participation seems an essential element. Nevertheless, outside the United States, birth control is not always a voluntary choice. In China, for example, Deng Xiaopeng initiated a "one-child" policy as a radical solution aimed at reducing the country's billion-person population. Couples can be fined and women pressured to abort or be forcibly sterilized if they violate the rule. Exceptions exist in rural areas, but since 1979 the policy has been rigidly enforced for most ethnic Chinese couples living in urban centers.

Most Americans do not fear a Chinese-style family planning policy, but the question of voluntariness is not always clearly defined. Federal funding obscures the line of authority between a woman's right to become pregnant and the government's right to control its population. Since the earliest origins of the birth control movement, some advocates have called for more proactive controls on population growth. When combined with a hierarchical theory of race, the move to check natural growth rates led to eugenicists targeting "dependent" populations in order to guarantee

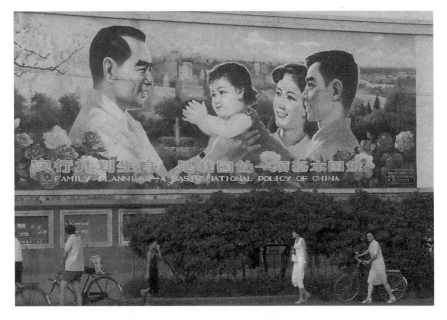

People walk past a billboard encouraging couples to have only one child. The one-child policy, as it is known in the Western world, refers to the controversial regulations concerning birth control in China. (Corel)

a stronger race from among the "better" populations. Margaret Sanger supported the eugenics movement, and prior to World War II, most advocates of birth control used eugenics arguments to justify broad legalization.

After the war, race-based eugenics arguments were irreparably tainted by Hitler's attack on Jews and other non-Aryans that resulted in the systematic murder of almost 10 million people during the war. By the 1950s, most birth control advocates reframed their eugenics arguments to focus on overpopulation rather than race. In the process, they successfully linked fears of Cold War deprivations with the threat of unregulated population explosions in Africa, Asia, and South America. By the 1960s, many Western countries spent millions of dollars in foreign aid for family planning programs intended to fight conditions that could lead to Marxist revolutions. Ending unwanted pregnancies was viewed as a necessary step to reducing poverty levels. Since the targets of these efforts lay overseas, most Americans were either supportive of or ambivalent to the efforts.

Yet the similarity in results was difficult to overlook. When President Johnson allocated federal money for family planning as part of his war on poverty in 1968, there were some critics who could not distinguish between the Cold War measures aimed at overpopulation and the earlier eugenics programs aimed at cleansing public health by preventing procreation of those deemed "unfit." In both cases, the government organized programs to reduce the number of new children born to "dependent" groups. Many black civil rights leaders, including Malcolm X, Bobby Seale, and Jesse Jackson, criticized family planning as a solution to urban poverty, warning that when birth control is directed toward a specific group, it amounts to a kind of "race suicide."

During the first decades of the twentieth century, eugenicists openly advocated for the sterilization of criminals, epileptics, and the "feeble-minded." Race could not be specified in law, but advocates pointed generically to "dependents" who were comprised mostly of poor immigrants and other minorities. By the 1920s, more than half the state legislatures enacted and implemented eugenics sterilization laws allowing certain government authorities (such as mental hospitals) to forcibly sterilize individuals deemed unfit for reproduction. The Supreme Court affirmed the constitutionality of these state laws in *Buck v. Bell* (1927). These laws remained on the books and in some cases in practice throughout the 1960s and 1970s.

By law, race was not supposed to be factor when deciding involuntary sterilization. Nevertheless, as late as 1965, the ratio of sterilization was twice as high for black women as it was for white women. Since minority groups, such as African American and Latino populations, were disproportionately represented among the urban poor, some critics interpreted the family planning programs as an assault against minorities. When anti-poverty advocates referred to "low-income households" needing to reduce their numbers to protect the health of society, some civil rights leaders feared ulterior motivations based on race-based eugenics. Within the black community, efforts to promote birth control were often ignored as a tacit effort to weaken their numbers.

This resistance intensified in 1973 after *Ebony* magazine published an exposé on young women in poor neighborhoods, some as young as 12 years, who underwent sterilization procedures without their knowledge or the consent of their parents. In some cases, the parents of young teens were asked to sign release forms but were told that they were for vaccinations or "shots." The children were then taken back into surgery where they underwent tubal ligation procedures. In other instances, pregnant women in small towns claimed that local doctors worked in conjunction with community-based family planning clinics to pressure them to accept sterilization. The doctors colluded to deny their delivery services unless the mothers agreed to tubal ligation after the birth.

In the 10 years after President Johnson's war on poverty, estimates suggest that more than 1,000 women were sterilized without their full consent. Most of them were African American, and all were on public assistance programs. During the Nixon administration, the federal government increased funding for voluntary sterilization procedures as part of the Medicaid health care. Federal law required informed consent, but the policy was difficult to enforce if other social pressures were included, particularly in small rural towns.

Supporters argued that those who accept state aid and welfare should expect to follow state guidelines. In 1973, 14 states considered resolutions to attach sterilization requirements to state welfare provisions. The American Civil Liberties Union filed several lawsuits, and no state legally permitted involuntary sterilization on the basis of income. Nevertheless, throughout the 1970s and 1980s, the African American community remained largely suspicious of family planning programs, fearing that they might be a modern form of eugenics-based racism.

LONG-ACTING CONTRACEPTIVES AND VOLUNTARINESS

The question of involuntary sterilization extends beyond federal mandates. Recent advances in contraceptive technology cause some critics to fear a modern equivalent to involuntary sterilization similar to that practiced during the 1930s. The Food and Drug Administration (FDA) approved a redesigned intrauterine device (IUD) that could remain in place for years at a time. These long-acting birth control devices were marketed as a convenience for women who did not want to take daily oral contraception. Many family planning doctors, however, also saw the device as an effective way to guarantee more population control by ensuring fewer opportunities for women to change their mind about using birth control.

The historian Rebecca Marie Kluchin recounts a letter written by Alan Guttmacher in the 1960s in which he praises the new IUD because it was "cheap" and because, once inserted, "the patient cannot change her mind. In fact, we hope that she will forget that it is there and perhaps in several months wonder why she has not conceived." Many family planning advocates of the 1960s and 1970s were strongly motivated by a goal to reducing the population. One of the greatest obstacles to achieving genuine population growth was that women change their mind. Long-acting contraceptives reduce the need for daily decision making, making the original decision to avoid pregnancy much more enduring.

Unlike sterilization, IUDs are rarely inserted involuntarily. During the 1960s and 1970s, when the cases of involuntary sterilization were most common, the procedures of tubal ligation were performed under general anesthesia, making it possible that a patient could unknowingly undergo such an operation, particularly if the patient was young and uneducated. By contrast, IUDs must be inserted by a physician in the woman's uterus through the vagina, so it is unlikely that a patient would be unaware of its presence. Women must at least initially agree to the initial insertion. But, as Guttmacher predicted, the question of voluntariness comes at the point of extraction. Modern IUDs can remain in position for years at a time, so contraception remains the default condition until the woman makes a deliberate appointment with a doctor's office to have the device removed. If the woman chooses to do nothing or simply forgets, then she will be effectively sterile.

Since the 1990s, the requirement of a patient's initial acquiescence was questionable after new technologies were developed that made it possible for a women to enter a doctor's office to receive a "shot" and then leave without knowing that she had been given a long-acting contraceptive. In 1992, the FDA approved Depo-Provera as an injectable contraceptive that remains in a woman's system for up to three months. Manufacturers developed the product in the 1960s and made it available to women in developing countries almost immediately. This practice later revived questions about the relationship between overpopulation theories and race-based eugenics since, as critics argued, American organizations willingly used the untested product on poor women overseas, even though it was illegal for women in the United States.

In fact, however, Depo-Provera was being used in the United States as well. The manufacturer, Upjohn, used the drug on an experimental basis through a network of publicly funded family planning clinics in mostly African American neighborhoods around Atlanta for 11 years. Later examination of procedures revealed that patients were not always fully informed of what they were taking, nor were they warned of the potential side effects. Other results indicated that cervical cancer rates among test subjects were significantly higher than the general population and included some fatalities. Critics argued that poor women were being unjustly experimented on because their populations were unwelcome in society. Since 2005, several large class-action law suits have been filed in relation to unadvertised side effects of Depo-Provera, including increased risks of osteoporosis.

Even without the abuse of ill-advised research methods, the question of voluntariness follows all long-acting contraceptives. The drug Norplant was developed in 1990 as a slow-release contraceptive agent contained within six small silicon rods that are implanted just below the skin, usually on a woman's upper arm. Although the initial insertion was more intrusive than a single "shot," it was much simpler than the extraction, which was a much more delicate procedure. The device could be effective for five years, but the side effects of Norplant were so severe (headaches and excessive bleeding) that most women chose to remove the implants after only three years. The difficulty of extraction raised questions about whether the sterilization was indeed temporary.

Norplant was discontinued in 2000, but in 2009 a redesigned version of the same drug set was released under the name Inplanon. It uses a slow-releasing hormone called etonogestrel, which is contained within a single silicon tube. It is effective for three years and slightly easier to remove. Long-term effects are yet to be seen, but critics contend that the question of voluntariness is inherent with any long-acting contraceptive alternative.

Also in the 1990s, lawmakers in several states submitted bills attaching family planning provisions to their welfare plans. Rather than force involuntary sterilization, the new approach provides financial incentive to achieve the same result. The proposals recommended additional benefits for recipients who agreed to take a long-acting contraceptive, such as Depo-Provera or a Norplant equivalent. Lawmakers recognized that daily contraceptives require daily decisions to continue to take them, but long-acting contraceptives remove those daily decisions from the patient. The Supreme Court has not weighed in on the question of whether the state's right to promote family planning outweighs an individual's right to procreate. The question remains highly controversial.

VOLUNTARINESS: DOCTORS AND THE "CONSCIENCE CLAUSE"

The proposed linkage between welfare and family planning is not without precedent. Government funding always provides opportunities for new regulations into areas of private life that would otherwise lie outside state jurisdiction. If the public is going to pay for an entitlement, then the state has a right to place restrictions on how the entitlement is used. The $300 million budget for Title X programs entitles the federal government to stipulate numerous conditions on their implementation. Yet $300 million pales in comparison to the $688 billion that the federal government spends on Medicare/Medicaid health insurance programs every year. That amount of money opens the way for a great deal of federal oversight of how hospitals, pharmacies, physicians, and insurance providers are reimbursed for their services.

The companion issue to involuntary contraception imposed on patients is whether doctors can be similarly compelled to provide birth control when it goes against their personal convictions. In 1999, the FDA approved an emergency conceptive drug containing levonorgestrol, which, when taken in two doses 12 hours apart, within five days after sexual intercourse, was 75 to 89 percent effective in preventing pregnancies. The "morning-after" pill was marketed under the name "Plan B" and immediately became a source of controversy related to voluntariness of health care providers. Some federal lawmakers proposed bills that would guarantee access to emergency contraceptives for rape victims.

Emergency contraceptives are controversial by nature because researchers are unable to determine if they act as contraceptives or as abortifacients. The evidence is inconclusive, and as a result many Catholic doctors and Catholic hospitals refuse to prescribe or provide the drug because of religious convictions. Some lawmakers argued that denying women access violated their right to complete health care, which was a more pressing need than individual conscience. The resulting federal bill would have applied equally to public and private hospitals, including Catholic hospitals that are morally opposed to the drug.

Federal lawmakers failed repeatedly to find votes for passage, but since 1999, 16 states have passed similar bills requiring health care facilities to either provide information or initiate procedures for women to come to such facilities after a sexual assault. The issue became more controversial as emergency contraceptives became more available.

In 2005, the FDA considered whether to approve the sale of Plan B without a prescription. Pharmacies around the country indicated that they would not carry the drug, triggering another national debate on whether health care providers can choose not to provide certain services on the basis of moral or religious grounds. Family planning advocates argued that failure to supply contraceptives on demand amounted to sexual discrimination. In 2006, the FDA approved over-the-counter sales of Plan B to women over the age of 18, and some Democratic lawmakers immediately responded with new bills requiring pharmacies to carry all contraceptives, including emergency drugs. Federal legislation failed to win approval, but seven states passed **Guaranteed Access to Prescription** laws, which force pharmacies to fill all prescription, including contraceptives.

Coming from the opposing side of this issue, many physician groups lobbied for specific federal protection from these legal consequences. These **conscience clause** proposals reflect a history of similar provisions stemming from the legalization of abortion. In 1973, Congress passed the "Church Amendment," which prohibited state or federal lawmakers from forcing doctors, hospitals, or other health care providers to perform abortions or provide facilities so that others could perform them as a condition of accepting federal money. By 1978, almost all state legislatures followed with similar provisions related to state funds. In 1988, Congress passed the Danforth Amendment, which clarified that hospital and other health care facilities could not be liable to sexual discrimination suits for failing to provide abortion services. Similar conscience clause laws were passed in 1996 and 1997, extending protections to medical insurance companies.

In 2009, Congress passed a new federal conscience clause provision that extended protection to doctors, pharmacies, and other health care entities that refused to provide contraceptive services on moral or religious grounds. The federal provision, however, does not necessarily override the existing state laws, which require the same groups to provide contraceptives on demand. The question was brought up routinely during the 2012 election cycle, and has not been fully resolved.

OTHER FACTORS: FOREIGN AID, ENVIRONMENTALISM, AND YOUTH

The federal government spent money on contraceptives for foreign nationals before it allowed funding for domestic clinics that serve Americans. This practice arose during the Cold War, when birth control advocates warned that the population explosions in Africa, Asia, and South America could threaten national security by creating economic conditions that were conducive to Marxist revolution. The modern version of this argument is that population explosions in developing countries could create an overdependence on industrial manufacturers that pollute and disturb the environmental balance of the earth.

Regardless of the explanation, a larger ethical question rises about the relative value of one population group over another. Why should poorer countries overseas or poorer communities in the United States be denied equal opportunity to procreate? Government-sponsored family planning programs almost always target the poor. Supporters argue that the people in those groups are in most need of government aid and therefore most affected by unintended pregnancies. Critics argue that the government's pressure not to procreate is more difficult to resist among those who are least empowered in society. At what point does family planning cease to be an issue of guaranteeing women the right not to have children and instead become a government imposition pressuring women not to conceive or propagate?

Included in this concern is the question of whether government-sponsored family planning programs are directing too much influence on youth education programs. It is difficult to distinguish between education programs to promote the public health and indoctrination programs to promote birth control as a solution to global population expansion. When do these programs overstep the boundaries of personal and religious convictions of each family? How can families who oppose birth control protect their children from education programs that are geared toward contrary conclusions? These and other questions are discussed more thoroughly in the next chapter, which discusses the social challenges posed by the widespread use of birth control in society.

CHAPTER 6

Social Impact of Birth Control

Advances in artificial birth control continue to inspire significant social changes in American culture and society. Since the late 1800s, the issue evolved from a question of decency into a matter of religious freedom, into a dilemma for public health, into a matter of scientific innovation and consumer protection, and, finally, into a mandate of civil rights, the empowerment of women, and environmental responsibility. Each successive development coexisted alongside its earlier incarnation, thereby expanding birth control into a far-reaching and relevant cultural question on many fronts.

Over the past 50 years especially, the prevalence of easily accessible birth control has played important roles in social relationships, particularly through the sexual revolution, the rise of feminism, and internecine conflicts among Christian churches (especially within Catholicism). Similar changes occurred politically, with contraceptives providing a means of federal expansion into private health care policies through newly reformulated population theories. Economically, oral contraceptives triggered the birth of a new pharmaceutical industry, inspiring both innovative marketing incentives and, unintentionally, a new field of civil litigation within the auspices of consumer protection. Considerable debate remains as to whether these changes are positive, negative, or morally neutral.

It is very unlikely that public access to artificial contraceptive methods and devices will be restricted in the near future—either legally or through social pressure. The historical evidence suggests that future trends will promote even greater expansion of access, practice, and government protection/funding. Nevertheless, the historic debates are far from dead. Birth control remains a dynamic public issue largely because it plays such a pivotal role in a diverse array of deep-seated ideological positions, including Catholicism, feminism, Malthusian population theories, and environmentalism. The use of birth control as a social policy will continue to inspire public debate because both advocates and opponents rely on deeply held views that do not easily accommodate compromise or consensus.

BIRTH CONTROL AND FEMINISM

A former president of Planned Parenthood, Gloria Feldt, explained in a 2006 interview that "when you peel back the layers of the anti-choice motivation, it always comes back to two things: what is the nature and purpose of human sexuality? And second, what is the role of women in the world?" She added that birth control was essential to women's rights because "if you can separate sex from procreation, you have given women the ability to participate in society on an equal basis with men." This is

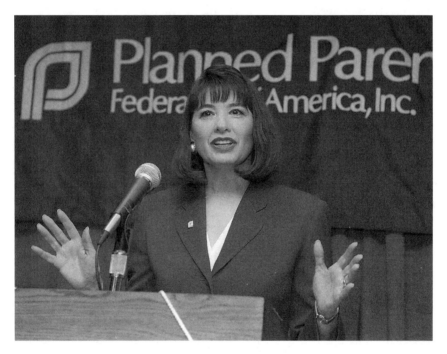

Gloria Feldt announces her new role as president of Planned Parenthood Federation of America at a 1996 press conference. Planned Parenthood provides family planning services for most state and federal government programs and in recent years has fought to remove all governmental limitations on abortion. (AP/Wide World Photos)

essentially the same view argued by Margaret Sanger in the 1910s and the same as that argued earlier by suffrage activists such as Elizabeth Cady Stanton in the 1870s.

Put simply as a generalized ideal, "feminism" is the belief that men and women should share equality in all aspects of life, including politics, economics, and culture, and that the opportunities available for men should also be made available for women. Beyond this simple definition, however, lay a wide variety of feminist ideologies regarding the sources for existing inequality and the best solutions for redressing that imbalance. Modern liberal feminism grows out of a Marxist dialecticism that presupposes three points: (1) men and women do not share common interests, (2) men currently dominate society through an industrial infrastructure designed to preserve their power, and (3) true legal, social, and economic equality is impossible without dismantling the existing social institutions. There is, of course, a broad spectrum of views between the simple ideal and the dialectical extreme.

From the perspective of most modern feminists, birth control is critical to women's emancipation from a male-dominated society because it severs the tie to childbearing. With contraception (and access to abortion if contraceptives fail), a woman can enjoy the same sexual freedom, economic independence, and political autonomy as a man. Liberal feminists further argue that men who oppose birth control do so precisely because they do not want to sever the biological tie that holds women to less active lives of domesticity. In this view, male-dominated institutions, such as the Catholic Church, reinforce the bonds of motherhood in order to keep women oppressed and removed from active involvement in sociopolitical endeavors. As the feminist historian Linda Gordon explained in her 2002 book *The Moral Property of Women*, "Conflicts about reproductive rights are political conflicts; that even what appear to be technological developments and neutral social scientific surveys must always be understood in political context."

For modern liberal feminists, all conflicts are gender-based contests. But the struggle for "reproductive rights" (which includes birth control and abortion) is the "Mother Controversy" because it centers around the key to physical emancipation for women. Without the means to break the bonds of motherhood, women are incapable of the physical independence that men at all times enjoy. For this reason, there is always an ideological association with artificial contraceptives. Although political lobbyists avoid direct references to "women's rights" when they advocate for government subsidies of birth control, there is nevertheless an unspoken pressure among liberal feminists that birth control is essential to liberation. Similarly, liberal feminists might be willing to compromise on almost any other political issue except for birth control (and abortion) because they hold this issue as central to their political activism.

LACK OF MALE CONTRACEPTIVES

From the perspective of liberal feminism, birth control remains under-promoted and underdeveloped. Women have almost free access to contraceptives, but feminist ideology argues that the patriarchal social system is still geared toward male convenience with the result that women must bear the primary responsibility for contraception. In the past half century since the invention of oral contraceptives for women, there has been very little research and development for similar technology for men.

About 6 percent of men undergo surgical sterilization procedures (vasectomy), compared to nearly 17 percent of women (tubal ligation), which is a ratio of almost one to three. There may be a variety of reasons for the difference. The most obvious is that women are always physically affected by pregnancy, while men are not, and men may escape responsibility by leaving the relationship. Women may be more likely to consider permanently ending their ability to conceive, while men may not want to commit to an irreversible procedure when other avenues of avoiding responsibility remain viable. There are other psychological reasons as well. Men may fear their sexual appetite, or their endurance may suffer from the procedure. Or they may feel less masculine, though that may be equally applicable to women who fear that sterilization makes them less feminine because they are incapable of fulfilling maternal roles.

Other social reasons for male reluctance to undergo surgical sterilization may be that the easy access to condoms makes the procedure less necessary. Condoms are not as effective as vasectomies (85 versus 99 percent), but they provide added protection against sexually transmitted diseases (STDs) that vasectomies do not address. If a man is going to use a condom as an STD barrier, then the permanence of the vasectomy may seem unappealing.

The concern about STDs came to a height with the appearance of the AIDS epidemic. During the mid-1980s, French researchers identified HTLAV-III (later known as HIV) as the virus that caused acquired immunodeficiency syndrome (AIDS). The number of reported HIV cases rose from 600 in 1982 to more than 3,000 in 1983. As a result, the Centers for Disease Control and the National Institutes of Health launched a variety of research programs to address the growing epidemic. In the process, numerous public education programs were started by public and private organizations intent on explaining the disease and warning people how to protect against infection. The most frequent single recommendation was to promote the routine use of condoms.

One unintended effect of the HIV/AIDS epidemic was that condoms were redefined primarily as a barrier against STDs, with much less emphasis as a contraceptive. Women were encouraged to continue artificial methods of birth control (primarily intrauterine devices and oral contraceptives), while men were encouraged also to use condoms to prevent STDs—this practice became known as "safe sex." The result is that men rely more heavily on women to assume the burden of contraception, and this might encourage some men to pay less attention to the responsibilities that follow unintended pregnancies.

Some liberal feminists contend that the prevalence of condoms as a tool for sexual liberation stems from an absence of effective male contraceptives. The result is that women suffer the physical, psychological, and economic side effects of preparing for contraception, while men increase their autonomy with little or no concern about the consequences of their sexual activity beyond protection against STDs. This feminist argument contends that male contraceptives would encourage men to share more equally the responsibility and related burdens for contraception.

RECENT INNOVATIONS IN MALE CONTRACEPTION

Researchers in other fields have unintentionally made discoveries that could potentially result in a male oral contraceptive. In 2009, a research group at Oxford University examined the genetic makeup of sperm and isolated the PLC zeta protein, which may be responsible for male infertility. The goal of the research was to uncover some solutions to male infertility, but this discovery also unintentionally opened a new avenue into research on male contraceptives. Researchers might be able to develop a reversible male oral contraceptive if they could discover a drug combination that switched the PLC zeta protein on or off at will.

Another unexpected development in male contraceptives arose out of cancer research. Some male patients taking the drug Lonidamine for their chemotherapy treatments discovered that they were also infertile. The risk of liver damage rendered Lonidamine unsuitable as a routine male contraceptive, but researchers working with New York's Population Council began working on a related drug called Adjudin, which acts as a contraceptive by preventing sperm from reaching maturity.

There is also some direct research into nonhormonal-based male contraceptives. One intrusive method under development by researchers in

India requires an injection that covers the interior walls of the vas deferens with a solution that destroys the sperm cells as they pass by. Other areas of research include mechanical devices that kill sperm without the need for chemical treatments. Among the options considered are ultrasound devices that heat the scrotum, specialized underwear that forces the testicle inside the abdomen to overheat the sperm, and any combination of devices that use hot water to elevate the temperature of the scrotum. The long-term effect of these options has not been studied, and it is not clear if these methods are reversible.

Most of the research into male contraception has been funded by organizations driven by broader objectives of population control. There does not appear to be a significant demand for male contraceptives in the marketplace, and this explains why there has been comparatively little research-and-development money devoted to the product. Almost all male contraceptive options remain in the development phases.

ENVIRONMENTALISM AND BIRTH CONTROL

In addition to liberal feminism, the modern environmental movement also provides a strong basis of ideological support for modern family planning policies and generally promotes the widespread use of contraceptives. Environmental ideology arose indirectly from a combination of the Malthusian theories of the 1800s with a new form of conservationism arising in the early 1900s. The Malthusian theories predicted that high rates of population growth would inevitably outstrip available resources needed to support them. The conservation movement arose in reaction to the noticeable impact of industrialization on natural resources. The modern ecological environmentalism of the 1960s combines the concerns of overpopulation with related concerns for industrial pollution, resource depletion, and endangered species.

Early pioneers of ecological environmentalism were called conservationists because they hoped to conserve natural resources, which were being consumed, polluted, and otherwise destroyed by the expanding urban footprint of factories, mines, mills, and other by-products of an industrial economy. The priority of protecting nature from human influence distinguishes environmentalism from other neo-Malthusian movements (such as eugenics) because it depicts humanity more as a perpetrator than as a victim of future disasters.

Both neo-Malthusian eugenicists and ecological environmentalists support greater use of birth control, but they do so for different reasons. The first ideology seeks to limit population in order to facilitate a healthier human race, while the second seeks to limit population growth in the order to more easily manage humanity's impact on the planet's ecosystems. During the most of the last decades of the twentieth century, the two views worked closely together to promote family planning education and practice. The first signs of division occurred around the turn of the millennium.

In 1997, during a conference on global warming held at the White House, Vice President Al Gore said that it was time to get beyond the controversies of family planning in order to save the planet. While recognizing that birth control and access to abortion empower "women, socially political, and in the context of the family, to participate in the decisions about childbearing," Gore further added that family planning education and services also reduce the world's overpopulation. Fewer people would decrease global dependency on natural resources, thereby reducing the causes of global warming.

Gore's linkage between family planning and ecology came under a test shortly thereafter. Researchers in Washington State uncovered elevated levels of synthetic estrogen hormone in its local waterways, resulting in reduced fertility levels in male fish. The study prompted reactions from opponents of family planning, especially some Catholics, who argued that oral contraceptives were poisoning the nation's environment and its moral health. Some public commentators feared that the nation's favorite birth control method, oral contraceptives, was actually hurting the environment by poisoning the waterways with synthetic chemicals.

The question led some environmentalists to consider other birth control methods. In addition to progesterone-based contraceptives, latex condoms were also deemed a potential environmental hazard. Latex is not biodegradable, and most people dispose of their used condoms by flushing them down the toilet. Most wastewater treatment systems address organic matter only and have no mechanisms for synthetic materials, meaning that the condoms often find their way into larger waterways. If they pass into the oceans, they could potentially combine with other garbage to form giant rafts made of various plastic materials.

Some environmentalists responded with calls for nonchemical-based methods of contraception. The threat of overpopulation can be viewed as both an environmental issue and a eugenics concern, so a new search began for "green" contraceptives. The result was that many modern environmentalists discourage the use of hormone-based methods and instead recommend intrauterine devices or permanent sterilization.

The modern environmental movement provides another ideological motivation for the support and promotion of widespread contraceptive use. A variety of social movements may support the idea of birth control, yet that does not mean there is also peace among the various supporters. Environmentalists, neo-Malthusians, and liberal feminists may be united in their opposition to legal or social obstacles to birth control. Yet because the ideological rationales of each group differ, the assertion of specific policy recommendations and implementation strategies often require considerable public debate and compromise.

PLURALISM AND IDEOLOGICAL DIVERSITY

A very large majority of American women practice one or more methods of artificial birth control; the Guttmacher Institute estimates that 99 percent of all sexually active women have used at least one contraceptive method at one time or another. At any given time, 17 percent of women in their childbearing years use oral contraceptives, another 17 percent undergo sterilization through tubal ligation, and 20 percent use other mechanical means, such as a vaginal ring, an intrauterine device, or another long-term hormone delivery system (implant, patch, or injection). More than 25 million women currently use artificial methods, or roughly 41 percent of all women of childbearing age (15 to 44 years). When combined with male sterilization and condoms, the number jumps to over 90 percent of sexually active women.

Liberal feminists strongly support artificial birth control, but that does not mean that all women who use contraceptives are liberal feminists. There are fewer women who identify themselves as feminists than there are women who use birth control. National polls of the past 30 years indicate that a slight majority of women identify themselves generically as "feminists." Similarly, few women treat birth control and abortion as equally important issues in reproductive rights.

Polls over the past 20 years suggest that women were generally more likely to be pro-choice than pro-life, but those trends have seen a slight reversal in recent years. In 2009 and 2010, recent polls suggested that a slight majority of women opposed abortion for all reasons except saving the mother's life. The generic "pro-choice" label refers to support for legal abortion under certain limited circumstances (first 12 weeks or for reasons of mental or physical health). A much smaller minority, less than a quarter of women, believed that abortion should be legal in all circumstances. This is in stark contrast to the broad support for birth control in any circumstance.

Liberal feminists argue that abortion is a necessary recourse when birth control fails or is unavailable. This support for unrestricted abortion rights is a core premise of liberal feminism, yet only about 25 percent of women agree with it. That is only slightly more than the 20 percent of women who oppose abortion for all circumstances, except situations when a woman's life is in immediate danger. These numbers suggest a broad disparity between the number of women who base their support for birth control on feminist ideology and those who do so for other more practical, perhaps nonideological reasons.

A majority of women practice birth control. But there is only a minority of women who strongly identify with liberal feminism. Likewise, there is a minority of American women who oppose birth control and liberal feminism based on their religious convictions. There are also women who support birth control but reject the presumptions of liberal feminists. The ideological spectrum between those who unequivocally oppose birth control (such as traditional Catholics) and those who unequivocally support birth control for ideological reasons (such as liberal feminists) reveals a great variety of deep-seated convictions in between. These differences are perhaps more obvious on questions of abortion than they are on questions of birth control, but there is a variety, and it is not necessarily reflected in the broad uniformity of practice.

In a pluralist society, where men and women hold a variety of ideological perspectives, social policies must respect the legitimacy of minority and dissenting views. Our American society prides itself on our respect for civic pluralism, so the variety of ideological viewpoints related to birth control creates a dilemma for policymakers and educators alike. How do we discuss birth control in a pluralist society without dismissing one or more religious or philosophical positions? The traditional Catholic view may be a minority in American society, but so too is the modern liberal feminist view. The majority of women practice some form of artificial birth control, but they do so for a variety of reasons, some of which might be mutually exclusive. How can a pluralist society account for the deep-seated views of several opposing minorities?

FEMINISM AND MARKETING

There are some issues that liberal feminists and opponents of birth control can agree on. Common opposition exists toward certain marketing strategies used by pharmaceutical companies to advertise directly to consumers. Liberal feminists generally applaud the nonverbal marketing cues that accompany birth control ads. In television and print media, young women who use birth control are portrayed as thoughtful, intelligent, and independent minded. But the birth control ads on television also opened the doorway to other sex-related products that often objectify women as passive recipients of sexual attention. Liberal feminists join many conservatives in opposing the new direction of television ads that emphasize crass sexuality.

Since the mid-1990s, the Food and Drug Administration (FDA) has allowed direct-to-consumer television advertising as long as the pharmaceutical companies included adequate warnings of potential health risks.

This policy change was intended to offset another provision, which barred pharmaceutical companies from providing gifts and financial incentives directly to doctors as part of the company's marketing strategy. Instead, drug companies were forced to redirect their marketing directly to the consumer. The new approach raised questions of consumer liability. In 1999, the Supreme Court affirmed the legality of this practice in *Perez v. Wyeth*, which involved a consolidated civil liability claim against the distributors of the long-acting contraceptive Norplant. Among other issues, the Court recognized that massive advertising campaigns can create environments in which consumers are more likely to request a drug than they are to wait for a doctor to prescribe one. In this manner, drug companies do share some liability in falsely advertising their products. The ruling, however, also affirmed companies' right to market direct to the consumer.

By 2005, drug companies were spending $7.5 billion on direct-to-consumer advertising. Lawsuits continued to be filed, including a major class-action suit against the leading brand of oral contraceptives, Yaz, which claimed to cure acne, mood swings, and menstrual irregularity. But the door had been opened to legally advertise prescription medication on any broadcast medium, and the advertising has been successful. Surveys of doctors in 2002 and 2003 indicated that 92 percent of their patients requested specifically advertised drugs.

In 1999, Pfizer launched a small television ad campaign for Viagra, which treats erectile dysfunction. In the advertisement's initial launch, the term "erectile dysfunction" was never mentioned. By 2003, there were three competing products for the disorder, and the advertising became increasingly more competitive and more explicit. Not only were there sterile phrases like "erectile dysfunction," but other terms and nonverbal cues directly related to sexual satisfaction and endurance were included as well. Images of a sterile doctor's office were replaced by images of men and women in the bedroom with overtly sexual messages.

These shifts in tone of the new commercials opened the way for other products that were more openly sexual in nature—without any pretense of scientific objectivity. Some of these included new television ads for sex toys (vibrators), websites selling personal introductions for anonymous sexual encounters, and several different companies advertising herbal supplements for "male enhancement" that promised to increase penis size. By 2010, television advertising for sex-related products reached several billion dollars.

Feminists and conservatives alike complained that new sex-related advertising targeted mostly male consumers and as a result usually depicted women as sexual objects with no ambition beyond servicing male sexual desires. Liberal feminists feared that the projected image of women not only reduced them to a level of male playthings but also encouraged women to participate in the condescension. For completely different reasons, moral conservatives criticized the reduction of sexuality to a matter of entertainment, with no accountability and no expectations for long-term commitment. Both sides agree that the marketing promotes an unrealistic ideal that equates physical beauty with sex appeal, lifetime success, and general happiness.

Beginning in 2009, lawmakers from both parties considered legislation that would limit the hours during which sex-related advertising could be shown on publicly regulated television. The debate stirred up deeper issues—feminists and moral conservatives may have shared opposition to the trends, but they did not agree on the proposed solutions. The main point of contention was over the role that contraceptive advertising had on promoting or encouraging the other sex-related products. Conservatives wanted to limit all sex-related advertising, including birth control ads, to evening hours that cater to adult audiences. By contrast, feminists called for even more birth control ads to offset the irresponsible messages that come from the male-oriented sex products. Other lawmakers feared that any regulation on sex-based ads could lead to regulations on birth control itself on the basis of public decency and would inevitably open the path to other moral-based restrictions in public and sex education. Regulating one medical industry on obscenity standards necessarily invites regulations of other related products by the same rules.

The earliest prohibitions against birth control were based on generalized concerns for public decency and the need to protect public morality. During most of the twentieth century, advocates for birth control fought successfully to reframe the public debate on contraception from a question of decency to an issue of public health. Since the 1960s, both birth control and family planning played a role in dismantling the public sensitivity to obscenity and indecency, helping to normalize discussions of human sexuality as a matter of public health. Yet the new prevalence of sex-related advertising on television unintentionally resurrected long-dormant debates about the impact of birth control on public decency and morality. The role that birth control plays in this new growing social dilemma is still under debate.

YOUTH APPROPRIATENESS AND ADVERTISING

An added dimension to the problem of hypersexualized advertising is the question of age appropriateness. On average, children are exposed to 3,000 marketing images every day, including advertisements in bill-boards, in print, on the Internet, and in broadcast media as well as other less explicit methods of product placement, endorsements, and infomercials. At what point is a child capable of the intelligent discernment necessary to distinguish between legitimate instruction, qualified news, and blunt adver-tising? The issue is important because direct advertising bypasses the natu-ral filters of parental oversight. Many parents are concerned that the advertising can undermine their personal child-rearing goals.

Advertising for birth control becomes especially controversial when directed toward younger consumers. In 2001, Bayer HealthCare introduced a new synthetic progestin called drospirenone, which was combined with ethinyl estrodiol and marketed under the name Yasmin. The new drug com-bination was expected to reduce some of the uncomfortable side effects that were typically associated with oral contraceptives, including weight gain, abdominal aches, and premenstrual moodiness. Drospirenone decreases salt levels, causing the bloating-related ailments. It also contains **antimi-neralocorticoid** and **antiandrogenic** properties that block male sex hor-mones, and this can lead to acne. In 2007, the FDA approved Bayer's release of a modified version of the drug under the name Yaz, which was repackaged to enhance the natural acne-fighting properties.

Bayer launched a massive ad campaign for Yaz, which specifically tar-geted teens. Ads were placed in teen magazine, teen-oriented websites, and teen-oriented television programming. Birth control was only one of three FDA-approved uses for the drug, and it was also approved for pre-menstrual dysphoric disorder and acne fighting. The ad campaigns always mentioned the contraceptive use but often placed greater emphasis on pre-menstrual dysphoric disorder or acne fighting in order to distinguish itself from its competitors.

Unfortunately, drospirenone also increases potassium levels, and this can result in dangerous complications for women who already have liver or kidney problems. Particular threats included risk of developing thromboembolism, which is a blood clot that forms inside veins found deep within the body. Numerous complaints were filed with the FDA charging Bayer with misleading advertising that failed to adequately warn consumers of potential health risks. Eventually, these complaints culmi-nated with formal grievances filed by the attorneys general from 27 states. In 2009, the FDA investigated the problem and later announced a settle-ment with Bayer, requiring the company to submit advertisements for FDA approval and further ordered the corporation to run $20 million in corrective advertisements. Class-action lawsuits were launched immedi-ately thereafter.

All oral contraceptives include side effects. What distinguished the Yaz/ Yasmin case was that the drug was specifically targeting ailments that were most common among teens and adolescents. Included among the consumer protection complaints were other, deeper ideological concerns about the appropriateness of marketing drugs that presume sexual activity among a demographic for whom sexual activity is almost always a risky behavior— not only physically but also emotionally and psychologically. Should corporations be allowed to utilize direct-to-consumer marketing strategies that exploit teenage insecurities in order to increase the demand for prescription drugs?

The FDA rebuked Bayer HealthCare for misleading advertising, but it did not offer any ruling on the appropriateness of targeting the underage demographic. Advocates for more expanded methods of family planning education applauded the new medium of contraceptive advertising because it further removed social stigma that might cause sexually active teens to be too embarrassed to ask for birth control. From this perspective, it is more important to prevent pregnancy than it is to limit teen sexuality.

Opponents of the new teen-themed marketing strategies argue that they encourage early sexuality by contributing to a cultural environment that presupposes sex as a normal and expected behavior for unmarried teens. This hypersexuality in teen culture deteriorates the value of monogamous relationships that are necessary for enduring marriages. These differences between the viewpoints of supporters and opponents are fundamental in nature and reflect a deep-seated diversity over the nature of marriage, sexuality, and the responsibility of society to monitor them.

BIRTH CONTROL AND SEX EDUCATION

Television commercials enter private households, but parents can choose to turn the programming on or off at their discretion. Most parents do not have such control over the messages that their children receive at school. As such, another facet of the age appropriateness of birth control concerns whether and how children should be taught about contraception during their sex education classes at school.

The mere existence of sex education programs in public schools is rarely controversial, as American schools have included some form of sex education since the late 1890s. The earliest programs focused on basic biological functions, with supplemental instruction on how to maintain moral lives despite the growing hormonal pressures of adolescence and young adulthood. Groups like the American Federation for Sex Hygiene and the American Vigilance Association were formed in the 1890s both to prevent the spread of venereal disease and to suppress the practice of

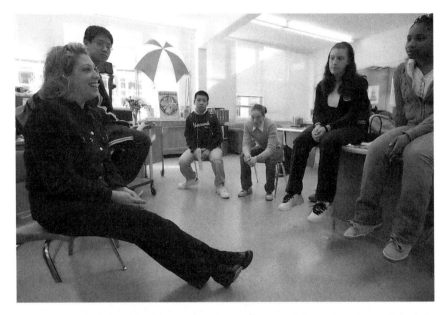

Ingraham High School health teacher Tamara Brewer, left, and students, from left, Alex Kon, 14; Tim Pham; Hannah Leifheit, 17; Kat McCarthy, 14; and DeKeira Wright, 14; give their impressions on the state of sex education in Seattle schools at Ingraham High School in 2006. Washington schools are not required to teach sex education, but in the districts where the topic does come up, between grades 5 and 12, state law mandates students be taught about abstinence but not about birth control pills or other ways to prevent pregnancy. (AP/Wide World Photos)

prostitution. Although rising from specific moral presumptions, the issue of sex education was treated as a public health concern.

By the 1910s, both associations merged together to form the American Social Hygiene Association (ASHA), which became the largest purveyor of sex education curriculum. The federal government got involved during World War I when increasing numbers of servicemen were coming home with debilitating sexually transmitted infections. Congress passed the Chamberlain-Khan Act (1918), which set aside federal funds for the sex education of men in the military, education that was produced mainly in conjunction with the ASHA.

Typical ASHA-based sex education programs identified the biological process, discussed the positive moral and physical benefits of abstinence outside a monogamous marriage, and then used detailed descriptions of syphilis, gonorrhea, and other common infections to demonstrate the harmful consequences of illicit sex. Public high schools began adding these programs in the 1920s and 1930s, and they became standard practice for most districts by the 1960s. With the exception of Catholic schools, there was little public controversy with the inclusion of sex education programs in public high schools until the 1960s.

In 1964, Planned Parenthood entered into the arena of sex education when it formed the Sexuality Information and Education Council of the United States (SIECUS). SIECUS was specifically formed to challenge the dominance held by ASHA in providing the curriculum for public sex education programs. Planned Parenthood's main concern was that existing curricula placed too much importance on abstinence and the prevention of STDs and not enough emphasis on the availability of birth control and the dangers of overpopulation. ASHA focused on sex education as a matter of public health, while SIECUS sought to use sex education curricula as a forum for promoting birth control.

CATHOLICISM AND SEX EDUCATION

Public conflict arises when schools teach birth control methods that reflect ideological presumptions contrary to those held by the parents. Should Catholic children be told that condoms and oral contraceptives are essential elements of safe sex? By contrast, should the children of unmarried parents be told that abstinence is the only healthy practice outside of marriage? The inclusion of birth control discussions within the context of sex education guarantees some public debate.

The Catholic Church opposed sex education from the outset, with a vocal opposition beginning in the 1890s and continuing until the 1960s. At that time, some dioceses in the United States began promoting a "Family Life" curriculum, which discussed the biological and moral aspects of sexuality. Following Pope Paul VI's encyclical *Humanae Vitae*, the U.S. Conference of Catholic Bishops issued an announcement in 1968 that affirmed "the value and necessity of wisely planned education of children in human sexuality." Since the 1970s, Catholic schools have included sex education programs that emphasize abstinence as a moral imperative outside of marriage.

Within the Catholic community, there continues to be great debate about the purpose and utility of sex education. On one side are those who argue that a "moral" sex education program is a necessary counter to the messages of modern sexualized society. On the other side are those who argue that any explicit sex education is immodest by nature and inappropriate for youth. Neither side supports instruction of artificial contraceptives, but advocates for sex education argue that students should be taught about natural family planning methods as an acceptable alternative to chemical birth control, while opponents argue that such instruction should be reserved for marriage preparation. Even within the confines of a specific ideological group, the question of how birth control should be taught to youth remains controversial.

Other controversies rise from the timing of sex education classes. Should schools develop a sex education curriculum for kindergarteners through high school seniors? Even supporters of including birth control information in high school sex education programs may hesitate to support sex education to five- and six-year-olds. The most common fear is that early exposure to sexuality desensitizes youth to eroticism and promotes a behavior that might otherwise remain dormant until later years. Yet supporters of comprehensive education argue that sexuality is a biological reality and that students need to be instructed from earliest ages on how to manage their sexual impulses in a way that does not lead to STDs, unintended pregnancies, or unnecessary abortions. The key difference between the two viewpoints is in how sexuality is viewed within a larger ideology.

Sex education became suddenly much more controversial in the late 1960s because students were being exposed to differing ideological approaches behind birth control. During the 1920s and 1930s, ASHA was dominated by an ideology that promoted abstinence as a tool for suppressing prostitution and vice. In the 1960s, Planned Parenthood was dominated by neo-Malthusian concerns about overpopulation. After the legalization of abortion in 1973, Planned Parenthood became increasingly dominated by liberal feminist ideologies that equated birth control (and abortion) with emancipation for women, young and old. Catholic ideology promotes sexuality as an exclusive property of marriage, intended primarily for reproduction. Each approach to birth control reflects a distinctive ideological view, and the diversity of views is directly connected with the level of controversy associated with birth control and sex education.

ABSTINENCE-ONLY SEX EDUCATION: NO BIRTH CONTROL

The federal government has dedicated money to family planning since President Johnson's administration. These Title X funds typically go to clinics that provide contraceptive services. Beginning in 2002, President George W. Bush launched a new federal program that set aside federal funds specifically for the teaching of abstinence as a primary means of birth control. During the eight years he was in office, funding gradually increased from $73 million to $204 million in 2008. Initially, most states accepted the federal money, though the program was politically controversial. After a publicity campaign launched by Planned Parenthood and the Guttmacher Institute, 17 states had by 2006 chosen to forgo federal funds in order to avoid abstinence-only programming.

Planned Parenthood and the Guttmacher Institute strongly opposed abstinence-only education as both impractical and potentially harmful to public health. They pointed to surveys indicating that more than half of high school seniors were already sexually active; therefore, teens were in the most need of information to prevent pregnancy and avoid STDs. Almost immediately, the Guttmacher Institute began gathering statistics to demonstrate the prevalence of teen sexuality and the subsequent increases in rates of teen STDs, unintended pregnancies, and abortions after the abstinence-only programs were initiated. The correlative data did not necessarily establish any causal connections, but the publicity campaign was very effective in encouraging new Democratic lawmakers in the 2008 Congress to reconsider the abstinence-only approach.

Perhaps a deeper objection for pro–birth control advocates was that the abstinence-only approach stigmatized teen sexuality and contraceptives, both of which have been promoted by Planned Parenthood as morally neutral. Catholics and other opponents of heightened sexuality within teen culture praised the abstinence-only approach precisely because it included some element, albeit unspoken, of moral judgment against premarital sexual relationships. It was that element of moral judgment that drew the strongest criticism from liberal feminists, zero-population-growth eugenicists, and environmentalists.

Federal sex education programs do not mandate any particular curriculum, but Congress can attach restrictions to federal money sent to states for sex education. The first federal grants that promoted an abstinence-only emphasis for federally funding sex education programs began in 1981 during President's Reagan's administration. The Adolescent Family Life Act (AFLA) provided funds for programs that discouraged premarital sexuality and promoted adoption instead of abortion when an unintended pregnancy occurs.

In 1983, the American Civil Liberties Union (ACLU) sued the federal government, arguing that AFLA grants went mostly to religious schools because they promoted religious presuppositions and as such was a violation of the constitutional mandate separating church and state. The argument was rejected by the Supreme Court in *Bowen v. Kendrick* (1988), which held that the state has a right to identify teenage sexuality as a public health problem and that religious institutions were uniquely positioned to help.

During President Clinton's administration, the AFLA program was altered to prohibit any specific religious references, with bans against holding AFLA-funded programs in religious sanctuaries. Funding was also reduced. It was against this background that President Bush launched the new abstinence-only funding bills. Like AFLA, most opponents used statistics to argue against what was mostly an ideological conflict. The debate remains largely politicized, with Democratic presidents generally supporting comprehensive sex education programs, which focus on birth control, and Republican presidents supporting abstinence-only programs, which do not.

The examples of AFLA and abstinence-only sex education demonstrate how public debate over birth control, which is already legal, can intensify when youth are included in the discussion. How can any single sex education program accommodate such diverse ideological positions without alienating or undermining alternative views? This question is difficult under any circumstance, but it is intensified by the fact that public schools deal with youth outside of direct parental control, and the prospect of indoctrinating children against the beliefs of the parents (and family) is always controversial.

BIRTH CONTROL ACCESS AND YOUTH RIGHTS

There are a number of influences that reach students within the school and yet remain outside the classroom and traditional sex education curricula. School health clinics or off-site clinics that receive referrals from the school workers may advertise, promote, and even distribute birth control to students outside of parental knowledge or control. These practices become controversial because of larger questions about the age at which youth can make intelligent decisions about their health needs.

The point at which the state deems children old enough to make their own medical decisions is called the **age of consent** and is determined at the state level. In 2010, 26 states and the District of Columbia contained laws allowing all minors age 12 and older to receive contraceptives without any parental approval. An additional 20 states allow only certain categories of minors to receive such services, and only four states have no laws governing the matter. Doctors in 18 states can prescribe treatments for sexually transmitted infections without parental knowledge or consent.

This issue is controversial and divides those who might otherwise approve of birth control for adults. Advocates argue that sexually active teens have the right to medical treatment that might lessen the dangers of their risky behaviors. Confidentiality helps to encourage teens to engage in safer sexual encounters and thereby prevents unintended pregnancies that affect the social welfare of the larger community.

Opponents argue that easy access to sex-related paraphernalia, including contraceptives, removes teens' expectations of personal accountability for their behaviors and only encourages sexual activity.

Complicating matters is the fact that the age-of-consent laws for voluntary sexual activity are not always the same as the age-of-consent laws for medical decision making. Most states set the age that a teen can voluntarily engage in sexual activity at 16—nine states set the age at 17, and 11 states use 18. Adults above the age of consent may be charged with statutory rape even if the sexual encounter was mutually voluntary. States may use a number of determinants to measure the severity of the crime, including the difference in ages between perpetrator and victim, the position of authority between the partners, and whether they are related by marriage.

The guiding principle behind age-of-consent laws is that teens below a certain age are not mature enough to make an intelligent decision about engaging in sexual activity. Adults who take advantage of youthful ignorance are charged with rape because teens are not old enough to knowingly agree to the encounter, and their innocence is being violated by an adult who should know better—even if teens think they know what they are doing. Twenty-six states set the age of consent for medical decision making at 12, yet no state sets the age of sexual consent at less that 16. Most states provide no provisions for sexual relations between teens of the same age, provided that they are older than 12, but there is always a penalty if one of the partners is a certain number of years older.

Some critics argue that there is a legal contradiction between laws that set the age of consent for medical decision making lower than the age of sexual consent. Teens are no better prepared to make decisions about their medical health, which includes birth control, than they are about engaging in sexual activity. If they are engaging in sexual activity below the age of legal majority, then the school or other public authority should inform the parents. Supporters of the lower age of medical consent counter by saying that the sexual activity between minors may or may not be legal and that medical confidentiality is more important than law enforcement. Again, the determining issue is whether it is more important to prevent STDs and unintended pregnancies than it is to monitor or prevent premarriage sexual activity.

PLURALISM AND MODERN SOCIETY

An important element of this debate is the question of whether the family should have more rights in protecting its own belief structure than the state has in protecting individual rights or the public's collective health.

Opponents of reduced-age-of-consent laws are part of a larger movement in the United States that describes itself as **pro-family**. Although not necessarily political, pro-family groups argue for laws that promote the family unit as the primary source of ideological instruction. Although nondenominational, specific issues—such as monogamous, heterosexual marriage; limited access to divorce; restricted access to abortion; and age-related restrictions on access to birth control and sex education—all reflect a distinctly religious worldview that is held by orthodox Jews, conservative Christians, and devout Muslims.

There is no "antifamily" movement, but the pro-family movement attracts opponents from a variety of issues ranging from liberal feminism to advocates of gay rights and zero-population growth. Collectively, these groups are often generalized under the **pro-choice** label, even though the particular issues are more broad based than support for abortion rights. Although not necessarily political, the pro-choice groups promote laws that emphasize individual rights over family obligations or family pressures.

Whether argued in the name of women's rights, gay rights, or youth rights, the opponents of the pro-family movement argue that individuals should not be restricted by constructed definitions of family rights. Liberal feminists argue that the traditional patriarchal family structure limits women's vocational opportunities and that laws should guarantee women the freedom to choose to have (or adopt) children inside or outside of marriage as they see fit. Gay rights advocates contend that laws based on the male-female definition of marriage limits equal rights of homosexual partners, and environmentalists argue that the emphasis on children in the traditional family definition promotes irresponsible population growth.

Birth control plays different roles for each viewpoint under the generic pro-choice label, but each group generally supports birth control as a necessary tool for individual emancipation and opposes restrictive legal or social pressures that are promoted in the name of family protection. These advocates argue that the state must assume more responsibility for protecting the rights that individual families may not recognize. Lower-age-of-consent laws, essentially, provide teens with legal protection to make decisions outside the knowledge or wishes of their parents. Confidential access to birth control allows women to practice contraceptives outside the knowledge or wishes of their spouse or partner. Advocates for the pro-family movement recognize the underlying purpose behind these laws and oppose them for the same reasons. They argue that the pro-choice ideology undermines the natural priority of family rights and deteriorates the primary parental role of educating their children.

There is no bright-line legal decision that can solve these types of conflicts. The fundamental difference in viewpoints is ideological and not based on scientific evidence for one view or the other. The pluralist nature of American democracy guarantees that advocates for both sides will continue to argue these points in the foreseeable future.

CONCLUDING THOUGHTS

There is no evidence of any strong public pressure to outlaw public access to birth control. There is, however, a great deal of public debate over how it should be paid for, how and when it should be advertised and taught, and the appropriate age at which birth control should be made available. These debates arise because they involve questions that reflect basic moral and ideologically differences. The controversies over birth control will continue to persist as long as American society continues to foster diversity of opinions.

The social impact of birth control can be measured by any of a number of diverse standards. Liberal feminists argue that oral contraceptives have empowered women, freed them from the bonds of motherhood, and provided the means for working toward greater equality with men. Neo-Malthusians argue that birth control has provided a necessary positive check to the constant population growth of the earth, thereby providing greater resources for a more intelligent and scientific structuring of society. Environmentalists point to birth control as one of many steps toward a general reduction in the human exploitation of the earth's resources.

In stark contrast, some Catholics or other similarly oriented religious groups point to the spread of easily available contraceptives as the start of a sexual revolution that objectified women, weakened the value of marriages, and led to a hypersexualized society with its concurrent problems of vice, addiction, and moral despair. Other pro-family groups recognize the usefulness of artificial contraception as an alternative to abortion but still lament the increasing sexualization of youth, the increase in divorce rates, and the general decline in moral accountability.

Obviously, there can be no easy reconciliation between the advocates and critics of the social impact of birth control. History has shown that the dominance of one ideological view may transcend others for a time but that it is rarely permanent. The dominance of the religious/moral view relegated birth control to the confines of obscenity during the 1800s and early 1900s. The eugenics/Malthusian view brought birth control out into open discussion as a public health issue during the 1930s. The rise of modern liberal feminism promoted birth control as a matter of civic rights in the 1960s. More recently, since 2000, environmentalism and concurrent fears of global warming have added a "green" dimension to the issue. Each generation adapts the dilemmas of birth control to the particular technological and social needs of its era.

History has also shown that the dominance of any single view does not eliminate the persistence of minority views. The Catholic Church maintains a strong opposition to artificial contraceptives on moral and religious grounds, while other pro-family groups oppose the expanded dissemination of birth control information and products for similar reasons. Yet, despite these and other criticisms among a minority of cultural voices, the larger majority of Americans continue to practice some form of legally guaranteed birth control. Trends suggest that the availability of and access to contraceptives will continue to expand even as the criticism remains relatively constant. As such, birth control will remain the center of dynamic social debate for the foreseeable future.

Primary Documents

Early Motivations for Birth Control—Part I: Science or Pornography?

EXCERPT FROM *FRUITS OF PHILOSOPHY*

Charles Bradlaugh and Annie Besant, *Fruits of Philosophy: A Treatise on the Population Question* (San Francisco: The Reader's Library, 1891), 5–9, 17–23, 24–26, 27, 40, 44–45, 51, 54–56, 72–77, 78–83, 84–85.

Charles Knowlton published Elements of Modern Materialism *in 1829. The book outlined his secular worldview, arguing that men were merely sophisticated animals, that there were no God and no soul, and that the religious feeling men sometimes feel "is nothing more nor less than a sensorial passion." He explained that "mankind are now too much enlightened to mistake mystification for explanation, or attribute effects to supernatural causes, when natural causes, amply sufficient to account for them, may be pointed out." Knowlton was a committed atheist who believed that the world could be entirely explained by science alone.*

As Knowlton expounded his atheist materialism, the rest of the nation was being swept up by the Second Great Awakening. This broad-based religious movement was inspired by a conviction that Jesus Christ was returning immediately and that the world had to be ready for him. The movement spread throughout the country, reaching its greatest intensity between 1829 and 1831. It was marked by camp meetings, religious revivals, and the rise of many new Christian denominations.

It was in the midst of this revival that Knowlton published The Fruits of Philosophy, *which was part birth control manual and part philosophy tract. His science reflected the limitations of the age, but this book was widely referenced at the time and was later exported to England, where it had a long life as part of the "freethinkers" canon of books.*

The following excerpt from The Fruits of Philosophy *provides an example of how Malthusian theories of overpopulation were used to justify the importance of birth control education as means of social reform. This excerpt also repeats the general list of birth control options that were typically recommended in manuals from the early nineteenth century before changes in rubber technologies made diaphragms and condoms more popular.*

FIRST.—*In a political point of view.*—If population be not restrained by some great physical calamity, such as we have reason to hope will not hereafter be visited upon the children of men, or by some *moral restraint*, the time will come when the earth cannot support its inhabitants. Population unrestrained will double three times in a century. Hence, computing the present population of the earth at 1,000 millions, there would be at the end of 100 years from the present time, 8,000 millions.

At the end of 200 years, 64,000 millions.
At the end of 300 years, 512,000 millions.

And so on, multiplying by eight for every additional hundred years. So that in 500 years from the present time there would be thirty two thousand seven hundred and sixty-eight times as many inhabitants as at present. If the natural increase should go on without check for 1,500 years, one single pair would increase to more than *thirty five* thousand one hundred and *eighty four* times as many as the present population of the whole earth!

Some check then there must be, or the time will come when millions will be born but to suffer and to perish for the necessaries of life. To what an inconceivable amount of human misery would such a state of things give rise! And must we say that vice, war, pestilence and famine are desirable to prevent it? Must the friends of temperance and domestic happiness stay their efforts? Must peace societies excite to war and bloodshed? Must the physician cease to investigate the nature of contagion, and to search for the means of destroying its baneful influence? Must he that becomes diseased be marked as a victim to die for public good, without the privilege of making an effort to restore him to heath? And in case of a failure of crops in one part of the world, must the other parts withhold the means of supporting life that the far greater evil of excessive population throughout the world may be prevented? Can there be no effectual moral restraint, attended with far less human misery than such physical calamities as these? Most surely there can. But what is it? Malthus, an English writer on the subject of population, gives us none but celibacy to a late age. But how foolish it is to suppose that men and women will become as monks and nuns during the very holiday of their existence, and abjure during the fairest years of life the nearest and dearest of social relations, to avert a catastrophe which they and perhaps their children will not live to witness. But, besides being ineffectual, or if effectual, requiring a great sacrifice of enjoyment, this restraint is highly objectionable on the score of its demoralizing tendency. It would give rise to a frightful increase of prostitution, of intemperance and onanism,[1] and prove destructive to health and moral feelings. In spite of preaching, human nature will ever remain the same; and that restraint which forbids the gratification of the re-productive instinct will avail but little with the mass of mankind. The checks to be hereafter mentioned are the only moral restraints to population known to the writer that are unattended with serious objections.

Besides starvation, with all its accompanying evils, over-population is attended with other public evils, of which may be mentioned, ignorance and slavery. When the mass of the people must toil incessantly to obtain support, they must remain ignorant; and where ignorance prevails, tyranny reigns.

Second.—*In a social point of view.*—Is it not notorious that the families of the married often increase beyond what a regard for the young beings coming into the world, or the happiness of those who give them birth, would dictate. In how many instances does the hard-working father, and more especially the mother, of a poor family remain slaves throughout their lives, tugging at the oar of incessant labor, toiling to live, and living to toil; when, if their offspring had been limited to two or three only, they might have enjoyed comfort and comparative affluence? How often is the health of the mother, giving birth every year to an infant—happy if it be not twins—and compelled to toil on, even at those times when nature imperiously calls for some relief from daily drudgery,—how often is the mother's comfort, health, nay, even her life, thus sacrificed? Or if care and toil have weighed down the spirit, and at length broken the health of the father; how often is the widow left unable, with the most virtuous intentions, to save her fatherless offspring from becoming degraded objects of charity, or profligate votaries of vice!

Nor is this all. Many women are so constituted that they cannot give birth to healthy, sometimes not to living children. Is it desirable, is it moral, that such women should become pregnant? Yet this is continually the case. Others there are who ought never to become parents; because, if they do, it is only to transmit to their offspring grievous hereditary diseases, which render such offspring mere subjects of misery throughout their sickly existence. Yet such women will not lead a life of celibacy. They marry. They become parents, and the sum of human misery is increased by their doing so. But it is folly to expect that we can induce such persons to live the lives of Shakers. Nor is it necessary; all that duty requires of them is to refrain from becoming parents. Who can estimate the beneficial effect which a rational moral restraint may thus have on the health and beauty and physical improvement of our race throughout future generations?

... A life of rigid celibacy, though infinitely preferable to a life of dissipation, is yet fraught with many evils. Peevishness, restlessness, vague longings and instability of character, are amongst the least of these. The mind is unsettled, and the judgment warped. Even the very instinct which is thus mortified assumes

---

[1]"Onanism" is a euphemism for masturbation, which comes indirectly from Genesis 38: 8–10.

an undue importance, and occupies a portion of the thoughts which does not of right or nature belong to it, and which, during a life of satisfied affection, it would not obtain.

In many instances, the genital organs are rendered so irritable by the repletion to which unnatural continency gives rise, and by the much thinking caused by such repletion, as to induce a disease known to medical men by the name of *Gonorrhea Dormientium*. It consists in an emission or discharge of the semen during sleep. This discharge is immediately excited in most instances by a lascivious dream, but such dream is caused by the repletion and irritability of the genital organs. It is truly astonishing to what a degree of mental anguish the disease gives rise in young men. They do not understand the nature, or rather, the cause of it. They think it depends on a weakness-indeed, the disease is on called a "seminal weakness"—and that the least gratification in a natural way would but serve to increase it. Their anxiety about it weakens the whole system. This weakness they erroneously attribute to the discharges; they think themselves totally disqualified for entering into or enjoying the married state. Finally, the genital and mental organs act and react upon each other so perniciously as to cause a degree of nervousness, debility, emaciation and melancholy—in a word, wretchedness that sets description at defiance. Nothing is so effectual in curing this diseased state of a body and mind in young men as marriage. All restraint, fear and solicitude should be removed.

... There have been several means proposed and practiced for checking conception. I shall briefly notice them, though a knowledge of the best is what most concerns us. That of withdrawal immediately before emission is certainly effectual, if practiced with sufficient care. But if (as I believe) Dr. Dewees' theory of conception be correct, and as Spallanzani's experiments show that only a trifle of semen, even largely diluted with water, may impregnate by being injected into the vagina, it is clear that nothing short of entire withdrawal is to be depended upon. But the old notion that the semen must enter the uterus to cause conception, has led many to believe that a partial withdrawal is sufficient, and it is on this account that this error has proved mischievous, as all important errors generally do. It is said by those who speak from experience that the practice of withdrawal has an effect upon the health similar to intemperance in eating. As the subsequent exhaustion is probably mainly owing to the shock the nervous system sustains in the act of coition, this opinion may be correct. It is further said that this practice serves to keep alive those fine feelings with which married people first come together. Still, I leave it for every one to decide for himself whether this check be so far from satisfactory as not to render some other very desirable.

As to the *baudruche*,[2] which consists in a covering used by the male, made of very delicate skin, it is by no means calculated to come into general use. It has been used to secure immunity from syphilitic affections.

---

[2]"*Baudruche*" is the French term for a condom made from animal skin.

Another check which the old idea of conception has led some to recommend with considerable confidence, consists in introducing into the vagina, previous to connection, a very delicate piece of sponge, moistened with water, to be immediately afterward withdrawn by means of a very narrow ribbon attached to it. But, as our views would lead us to expect, this check has not proved a sure preventive. As there are many little ridges or folds in the vagina, we cannot suppose the withdrawal of the sponge would dislodge all the semen in every instance. If, however, it were well moistened with some liquid which acted chemically upon the semen, it would be pretty likely to destroy the fecundating property of what might remain. But if this check were ever so sure, it would, in my opinion, fall short of being equal, all things considered, to the one I am about to mention—one which not only dislodges the semen pretty effectually, but at the same time destroys the fecundating property of the whole of it.

It consists in syringing the vagina immediately after connection with a solution of sulphate of zinc, of alum, pearl-ash, or any salt that acts chemically on the semen, and at the same time produces no unfavorable effect on the female.

In all probability a vegetable astringent world answer-as an infusion of white oak bark, of red rose leaves, of nut-galls, and the like. A lump of either of the above-mentioned salts, of the size of a chestnut, may be dissolved in a pint of water, making the solution weaker or stronger, as it may be borne without any irritation of the parts to which it is applied. These solutions will not lose their virtues by age. A female syringe, which will be required in the use of the check, may be had at the shop of an apothecary for a shilling or less. If preferred, the semen may be dislodged as far as it can be, by syringing with simple water, after which some of the solution is to be injected, to destroy the fecundating property of what may remain lodged between the ridges of the vagina, etc.

I know the use of this check requires the woman to leave her bed for a few moments, but this is its only objection; and it would be unreasonable to suppose that any check can ever be devised entirely free of objections. In its favor it may be said, it costs nearly nothing; it is sure; it requires no sacrifice of pleasure; it is in the hand of the female; it is to be used after, instead of before the connection, a weighty consideration in its favor, as a moment's reflection will convince any one; and last, but not least, it is conducive to cleanliness, and preserves the parts from relaxation and disease. The vagina may be very much contracted by a persevering use of astringent injections, and they are constantly used for this purpose in cases of *procidentia uteri*, or a sinking down of the womb; subject as women are to *fluor albus*, and other diseases of the genital organs, it is rather a matter of wonder that they are not more so, considering the prevailing practices. Those who have used this check (and some have used it, to my certain knowledge with entire success for nine or ten years, and under such circumstances as leave no room to doubt its efficacy) affirm that they would be at the trouble of using injections merely for the purposes of health and cleanliness.

. . . What has now been advanced in this work will enable the reader to judge for himself or herself of the efficacy of the chemical or syringe check, and time will probably determine whether I am correct in this matter. I do know that those married females who have much desire to escape will not stand for the little trouble of using this check, especially when they consider that on the score of cleanliness and health alone it is worth the trouble.

EXCERPT FROM *THE BOOK OF NATURE*

James Ashton, *The Book of Nature: Containing Information for Young People Who Think of Getting Married, on the Philosophy of Procreation and Sexual Intercourse; Showing How to Prevent Conception and to Avoid Child-Bearing; Also Rules for Management during Labor and Child-Birth* (New York: Brother Jonathan Office, 1865), 20–24, 42–46.

This second excerpt comes from James Ashton's The Book of Nature, *which was published at the end of the Civil War. Anthony Comstock identifies Dr. Ashton by name as an example of the kind of materials that he believed were presented as scientific manuals but that Comstock believed were actually thinly disguised pornography.*

The selection was included for two reasons. The first reason is to provide the reader with a specific example of the type of book that Comstock labeled as indecent. The second reason is to demonstrate the extent to which scientists knew about the reproductive process. Of particular interest are the assertions of an "energy force" connected to the sexual act. Despite the claims of neutral, scientific objectivity, most writers on the subject (both for and against) presumed a mystical and/or spiritual component to human reproduction. It is this supernatural presumption that most fuels the opposition to widespread education and practice of birth control.

The headings are original to the text.

The Philosophy of Sexual Desires

The sexual organs of man and woman are wonderfully adapted to each other, and have a perfect power of mutual attraction. Nature sacrifices every thing to reproduction: It is thus that we enjoy all strength, vigor and beauty, so as to excite us to contribute to the procreation of our species; and thus that such exquisite pleasure is associated with the copulative act. It is for this reason also that we experience so many sweet illusions in the brilliant season of our amours, and that we give way to others when our reproductive powers have failed. In a word, Nature always regards the species, and never the individual; and whatever we may say or think of our superiority over inferior animals, we cannot conceal from ourselves the fact that, like the brutes, we are influenced in our unions by the pleasure of sexual intercourse. It is useless to deny that the majority of marriages which are apparently based on the sentiment called love, are nothing more than the result of an involuntary obedience to the imperious voice of our sexual organs. A man admires the graceful figure, the voluptuous form, and the general female graces of a woman, and he at once desires to possess her person. This induces him to cultivate her acquaintance, and unless he finds something in her disposition positively disagreeable, ten to one he will offer her marriage. Who will deny that sexual desire was the moving cause of this connection? A woman meets a man of fine figure, noble gait and manner, broad chest, and elevated head, furnished with a luxuriant growth of hair. His eyes are full of fire, and he is amiable, gallant and polite. She at once feels a thrilling desire to become better acquainted with him. What is that but a sexual yearning? Thus far, certainly, no sentimental collusion can have occurred between them.

The philosophy of sexual desires has been frequently discussed by learned men, and interesting experiments have been made to test whether the attraction of the two sexes was not precisely the same in human beings as in the minor animals. These tests proved that our animal natures are not directed altogether by the intellect. We see young persons of opposite sex mutually caress and embrace each other by some mysterious influence, even before they are of sufficient age to experience sexual desires. This mutual attraction is attributed by some people to Animal Magnetism—the male being the positive, and the female the negative principle. We, however, believe it to be an instinctive sympathy; for experiments have been made which prove that the Generative Organs of either sex exercise a certain mysterious influence one upon the other. A French physiological writer says that two vigorous young persons were put in a semi-insensible state by the use of certain drugs. Being stripped and their private parts placed slightly in contact, (their heads being fully covered,) this slight touch instantly excited the sexual feeling. This experiment is reported in detail, and we do not doubt that it was *bona-fide*. The peculiar instinctive attraction in this case was so delicate that it acted almost like electricity to the male organ. Besides this instinctive attraction, the nervous sensibility is so constituted as to aid in the union of the sexes. In the present state of society, however, young people do not usually wait the slow process of Nature's teachings, but gain their knowledge by a precocious association or under the instruction of their seniors. The sexual impulse, under such circumstances, is forced and unnatural, and is frequently the parent of incurable disease.

Coition, or sexual union, may be compared to a fit of epilepsy, or to an electrical shock. It entirely engages both the mind and the body; we neither hear nor see, but the soul is entirely absorbed in the act. When a man is performing this act, if his thoughts wander, the product will be feeble, and if his wife become pregnant the off-spring will be inferior. This fact is applied to the offspring of great geniuses, who are supposed to be thinking of something else when they beget their children, and hence their descendants are often much below them in intellect. In further confirmation of this theory, history informs us that some of the greatest men the world ever saw were bastards—children begotten with vigor, and when the minds of the parents are supposed to have been absorbed in the one idea of a loving sexual embrace. Aristotle believed that the causes of deformed children, of monstrosities, and of all defective offspring, were in consequence of imperfect connections, or acts of generation when the minds of the parents were depressed by passion, anxiety, trouble, or any difficult or abstract matters.

Persons of moderate and regular habits, with strong and sound constitutions, beget healthful infants; while those whose habits are excessively mental, generally produce feeble offspring, though their constitutions and general health may be good.

Another cause of feeble children is the abuse of the function of generation by too frequent intercourse. In such cases the semen is thin and watery, being too suddenly secreted. Harvey says that to produce vigorous offspring, the spermatic fluid ought to remain two or three days in its receptacles for its thinner parts to become absorbed, when more vitality will be imparted to it, and hence the more vigorous will be the offspring.

It will be thus seen that the proper union of the sexes is at that moment when the mind and body are at rest, and when both parties are in a mood for mutual caresses. Certain moral and intellectual perceptions undoubtedly govern their feelings under such circumstances, and aid in producing that intense pleasurable feeling which a healthy and proper connection will always promote.

As to the times when sexual union should be avoided, I would say that during five or six days after the monthly turn of the female commences, it is absolutely unhealthy to both. Married men of cleanly habits will religiously observe the Jewish law in this respect, and wait seven days. It was formerly thought that connection with a female during the menstrual flow, was the origin of a certain sexual disease called gonorrhoea; but such is not the fact. Connection during that period is, however, unnatural, hurtful, and often painful to the female. Neither should there be any intimacy of this kind when the female is troubled with *fluor albus*, or whites, as then there is danger that the male may contract gonorrhoea. When a girl appoints her wedding day, she should reckon as near as possible a time when she will be fully over her monthly turn. If subject to *fluor albus*, she should first seek the most efficient means of cure; and if possible, a cure should be effected before she marries. Girls subject to this complaint seldom enjoy the constant sexual intercourse incident to married life. Medical science can manage this disease so easily and effectually by the aid of the Truss, or Abdominal Supporter, that there is no excuse for neglecting it. Unless the strictest cleanliness is practiced by the wife we she has the whites, she may give her husband the disease called gonorrhoea. She should never have any connection with him in the morning until she has risen and washed the part thoroughly. Suspicious men have often believed their wives unfaithful because they have contracted gonorrhoea from the whites. But the fact is well known to medical men that that alone is the original cause of the disease.

In Persia, and indeed in most Mahomedan countries where a plurality of wives is allowed, it is considered indecent to approach a woman for sexual intercourse during pregnancy, or when she is suckling her child. This custom is highly commendable, and if observed among Christians it would tend to promote the health of both the mother and her offspring, for Nature never intended that the nuptial act should be performed solely for the gratification of our passions. Nevertheless, I do not say that a moderate indulgence during pregnancy would be hurtful to a robust woman; though to a weak and nervous one it surely is. But after the child is born, sexual intercourse should cease until it is weaned, to insure its health. Many sucking children die in consequence of the sexual indulgences of their parents, and none are wholly unaffected thereby.

Effects of Too Early Sexual Intercourse

One of the greatest evils to mankind is a too free sexual indulgence by young men and boys. It not only injures their vital powers, but affects their intellects. Parents should watch their boys to observe whether they are of amorous temperament. If they are found to be so, a prudent person can find means to persuade or prevent their indulgence of sexual passion. If a boy is allowed free and habitual intercourse with females before he has attained his growth, it will not only prevent the full development of his body, but also of his intellect. This is a well known fact in physiology; and by this very means many youths, who would otherwise become distinguished, have settled down into mediocrity, with scarcely sufficient energy of character to earn a livelihood. In a certain family in one of the country towns on the Hudson River, three sons were born. The two oldest afterwards became distinguished men. It was a family that inherited naturally the fine talents of their father, combined with the extraordinary robust and nervous energy of the mother. It was impossible that such a couple could produce other than intellectual and vigorous offspring. The third son, up to the age of twelve or thirteen years, promised to be the flower of the family. His education was progressing favorably. He was the pride of his parents. Years rolled along, and it seemed as though the boy stood still at thirteen or fourteen. He was amiable, and learned his lessons weld enough, but all; the energy and fire of youth seemed to have vanished. He did not care to join in the manly sports of his elder brothers, but in a listless and dreamy mood preferred to stay at home. His parents began to have fears for his health, though he did not complain. The father finally took him to New York, and consulted a physician of eminence. The doctor asked some questions relative to his habits, but the simple and candid answers of the lad did not lead to anything explaining the real cause of his malady. At parting, the physician said to his father, that if the lad lived in New York, he should pronounce his case one of too early sexual indulgence, unless he practiced the silent vice of Onanism. "Are there no females is your neighborhood with whom the lad could by any possibility associate?," inquired the doctor. "He never goes in company at all," was the reply. "What servants have you?" "Two excellent girls who have been years in the family—the idea of an illicit association there is preposterous." His mother is positive that he does not practice the solitary habit?" "Yes!" "Well, I can do nothing for him; but yet I would like to see the boy again. With your permission I will run up to your place in a week or two." "We shall be happy to see you."

The doctor found out the secret of the boy's malady within twenty-four hours after his arrival. He had cohabited constantly with one of the maids from the age of twelve and a half years until he was sixteen! The lad was saved only because of his youth. He partially outgrew this severe shock to his nervous system; but yet never fully developed the intellectual powers with which Nature had endowed him. Young men who marry too soon are in the same category. There is not one in a dozen who is fully developed even at twenty-one years of age.

The case of the son of Napoleon I., Emperor of the French, was similar to that above related. At the age of fifteen or sixteen he began his career of sexual indulgence, which ended his life at the early age of twenty-one years. He, too, was an amiable, inoffensive and studious youth—beloved by his grandfather and by the whole Austrian Court; and though the son of the most energetic man that modern times has produced, yet, from his quiet and effeminate life, he scarcely attracted the least public attention.

The present Sultan of Turkey is a living evidence of the effects of too early indulgence in sexual intercourse. He is the son of a brave and vigorous soldier, and with proper culture would doubtless have become a great and good man. Abdul Medjid has been over twenty years on the Turkish throne, and has hitherto impressed those who came in contact with him simply as a weak and indolent young man, with good intentions, but with neither nerve nor energy to carry them out. It was generally believed, and with good reason, that in his ease, as in that of so many others of his race, the sensual indulgence begun in his boyhood had destroyed every trace of masculine decision. No one who watched his dreamy, listless expression, and saw his relaxed muscles, and lolling attitude as he rode on horseback through the streets, could help feeling that he reigned rather in virtue of foreign support than of his own ability to command obedience.

Results of Sexual Abuses

It was not our intention in this work to speak of Onanism and Masturbation. These unnatural practices are so generally known to be destructive to the sexual powers, and of health, that young people scarcely need advice on the subject. But it may be interesting to know the results of such practices, and of the abuse of the sexual organs by over indulgence. Some constitutions experience a sort of consumption which arises from the dorsal portion of the spinal marrow. No fever accompanies it, the appetite continues good, but the patient gradually wastes away. Women thus affected describe a crawling sensation down the spine. Men lose their seminal fluid in their urine, having a ringing in the ears, a weakness of vision, near-sightedness, and their intellectual capacities are weakened and confused. In short, the whole nervous system is generally prostrated. Excess of venery is likewise the first exciting cause of many painful diseases, such as rheumatism, neuralgia, epilepsy, convulsions, &c. Young married people are apt to indulge too much in sexual intercourse, and many a man lives a life of misery from ill health originated in this manner. Women are not affected so much by over indulgence as by Masturbation. Delicacy not allowing an ardent woman to tell her husband of her needs, she is apt to relieve herself by this unnatural practice. There are, however, but few women who crave sexual intercourse. The excess is generally on the part of the man. Moderation in sexual pleasures is the key to health in a great many cases where the patient is hopelessly lamenting his sad fate. Sometimes a man will indulge to excess with-out experiencing much inconvenience, when suddenly a fit of palsy or epilepsy prostrates him, and leaves him a hopeless invalid for life. I remember an interesting case in point. A man of robust health and strong sexual powers, married at the age of nineteen. From that time until the age of forty-five, he lived temperately, was regular in his habits, and never knew a day of sickness. He had always the reputation of being fond of a variety of women—indeed, this seemed to be the one passion of his life, for he dissipated a handsome property in settling crim. con. suits, and paying for bastard children. As he advanced in years his passion seemed to increase, and it was said that he supported five different mistresses at the time of the occurrence of the event I am now about to relate. One day when he was writing a letter, he felt a peculiar twitching of the forefinger with which he held his pen. This twitching sensation increased so much that he called on me for advice. I replied, "Let the women alone, for that is a symptom of palsy." Within two days thereafter he was struck down and lost the use of his hands, his right arm, and partially of his right side. Ten years have passed, and this man, who had previously enjoyed excellent health, is still as helpless as on the first day of his misfortune. He has consulted distinguished physicians—American, French and German—but there is no help for him. All agree that relief is impossible, but that he may live for many years an imbecile, palsied man.

To sum up: If you wish to maintain your intellectual faculties intact—to enjoy good health—to be cheerful in the decline of life—to keep your strength, your imagination, your memory, and your eye-sight unimpaired, refrain from too frequent intercourse with women. Once a week is quite often enough for this indulgence; and more than twice a week is positively hurtful. Some men may sneer at this advice, perhaps; but to such we say, look back upon your life. Are you as perfect, both physically and, intellectually, as you would have been had you curbed your sexual desires?

Early Opposition to Birth Control—Moral Temperance or Public Interference?

COMSTOCK LAW OF 1873

Congressional Globe, 42nd Cong., 3rd Sess., II (Washington, DC, 1873), 1240, 1307, 1436–37, 1525–26, 1571, 2004–5. *Statutes at Large of the United States of America*, 1789–1873 (17 vols., Boston, 1850–1873), XVII, 598–600.

The U.S. Congress passed the federal "Comstock Law" in 1873. Anthony Comstock represented a vocal constituency in New York City who feared that the growing urbanization was undermining America's moral values. The federal government was expressly forbidden to limit free speech and had no jurisdiction over local ordinances on decency. It did, however, have explicit jurisdiction over the postal system. In Article I, Section 8, of the U.S. Constitution, the federal government was given the power to "establish post offices and post roads." In 1878, the U.S. Supreme Court ruled in Ex Parte Jackson *96 U.S. 727 (1878) that Congress had the right to regulate any contents sent through the mail. This affirmed the constitutionality of the Comstock Law.*

Most states followed the federal example and passed similar laws, with specific details that reflected local interest groups. The Women's Christian Temperance Union created a special office dedicated to protecting the purity of women. They were largely responsible for pushing through state versions of the Comstock Law. It is relevant that literature relating to birth control was grouped together with abortion manuals and all other forms of pornography. Widespread acceptance of contraception did not become possible until that association was broken.

"An Act for the Suppression of Trade in, and Circulation of, obscene Literature and Articles of immoral Use."

SEC. 148. That no obscene, lewd, or lascivious book, pamphlet, picture, paper, print, or other publication of an indecent character, or any article or thing designed or intended for the prevention of conception or procuring of abortion, nor any article or thing intended or adapted for any indecent or immoral use or nature, nor any written or printed card, circular, book, pamphlet, advertisement or notice of any kind giving information, directly or indirectly, where, or how, or of whom, or by what means either of the things before mentioned may be obtained or made, nor any letter upon the envelope of which, or postal-card upon which indecent or scurrilous epithets may be written or printed, shall be carried in the mail, and any person who shall knowingly deposit, or cause to be deposited, for mailing or delivery, any of the hereinbefore mentioned articles or things, or any notice, or paper containing any advertisement relating to the aforesaid articles or things, and any person who, in pursuance of any plan or scheme for disposing of any of the hereinbefore-mentioned articles or things, shall take, or cause to be taken, from the mail any such letter or package, shall be deemed guilty of a misdemeanor, and, on conviction thereof, shall, for every offense, be fined not less than one hundred dollars nor more than five thousand dollars, or imprisoned at hard labor not less than one year nor more than ten years, or both, in the discretion of the judge.

EXCERPT FROM *FRAUDS EXPOSED*

Anthony Comstock, *Frauds Exposed* (Montclair, NJ: Patterson Smith Publishing, 1880 [1969]), 5–8, 388–94, 426–27.

Anthony Comstock traveled to Washington, D.C., in 1872 and gave testimony about the young lives he had seen ruined by the temptations of pornography. It was largely his testimony that secured the overwhelming support for the resulting decency act, which became known simply as the "Comstock Law." He was appointed special postal agent in charge of enforcing the new law and devoted the rest of his life to the suppression of vice. The following year, Comstock seized half a million books, pictures, and nearly 15,000 pounds of medicines marketed as aphrodisiacs. He was so successful that five years later, his office could find only 40 to 50 books and pictures per year.

The following selections were included to illustrate the larger temperance movement that fueled Comstock and similar champions of purity during the late 1800s. Comstock wrote Frauds Exposed *a half dozen years after his appointment as special postal inspector. He used the book to remind readers why his office was necessary as well as to answer some of his most vocal critics directly. In these excerpts, Comstock outlines many of the presumptions shared by his temperance supporters. How many of these presumptions continued to be held in the twentieth century? Do any of these presumptions continue to fuel support or opposition to contraception today?*

My object is to expose the multitudinous schemes and devices of the sharper to deceive and rob the unwary and credulous through the mails; to warn honest and simple-minded persons; to shield our youth from debauching and corrupting influences; to arouse a public sentiment against the vampires who are casting deadly poison into the fountain of moral purity in the children; and at the same time expose to public indignation the infidels and liberals who defend these moral cancer-planters. With malice toward none, but with unbounded sympathy and charity toward the multitudes who each year are defrauded through the mails, or cursed in mind, body and soul by obscene matter, I present some of the devices to plunder, ruin, and debauch, which it has been my privilege and duty to overthrow and stop, during a seven years' experience as a Special Agent of the Post-Office Department of the United States, and Chief Agent and Secretary of the New York Society for the Suppression of Vice. Let it be remembered, that these facts have been gathered in the discharge of my duty under my solemn oaths of office. Many of these are the evidences upon which juries have convicted and courts sentenced.

Another object is self-defense. Defense of my cause, first; and theft of my own good name. It is important that a man should be right in all he does: It is almost equally important, that he seem to be right when he is right. Many a time I have discharged my duty faithfully, accomplishing some very important object, or securing some notorious criminal dealing in vilest matters, and yet I have received nothing but misrepresentation, odium and abuse. One great difficulty that surrounds our work, is that we cannot publicly defend it with the facts. The facts cannot be published. Many persons sympathize with and defend those guilty of gravest crimes, simply through ignorance of facts, and condemn me because they are deceived by the prisoner's story; whereas, if they would but take one look at what we have seized in that very man's possession, they would ostracize the criminal. Prejudices have grown up, because of libels and slanders that have been printed in newspapers. I therefore, at the close, have presented one chapter where I put the truth beside the published slanders, and I ask a careful perusal of that chapter. I withhold the name of my defamer. I simply defend my cause, and my own good name, which is important to the successful prosecution of my official duties, by the presentation of the truth.

... But no part of this book can be of greater interest, than those chapters that expose the Liberal Fraud, and the infamous conspiracies entered into by the Liberals, to repeal the laws against obscene literature. I regret it becomes necessary to refer to some of these creatures. But when a body of men unite to advance a cause, which promises a morality better than that offered by the Word of God, a system of government better than the grand institutions of Free America, a religion purer and nobler than that of our Lord Jesus Christ; a hereafter more glorious than the eternal heavens, it is well for the public to know their true character. "By their fruits ye shall know them." I have presented facts; I have drawn an indictment against this horde of blasphemers and revilers of the ever-living God, and I submit my evidence to sustain this indictment. Let every decent man read, and see what we have in our land, and then say if they will consent that our youth shall be inoculated with this virus. Let youth read it, and then say if, in all this ranting mob, there is a character worthy to be placed before that of our blessed

Savior as an exemplar for them. Some have said: "You will be attacked by these fellows." My reply is, I cannot expect to have better treatment than our blessed Master. I stand by the record.

... This cursed business of obscene literature works beneath the surface, and like a canker worm, secretly eats out the moral life and purity of our youth, and they droop and fade before their parents' eyes.

This subject is one that none of us like to contemplate, and yet it is of most momentous consequence. When we stop and consider that the men and women of the next generation are to come from the boys and girls of to-day, we will find an unanswerable argument for keeping pure and good the youth and children of the present.

In 1872, when I undertook the great and all-important work of suppressing by legal process this hydra-headed monster, what did I find? I found a business systemized and systematically carried on. I found newspapers teeming with the advertisements of these bold and shameless criminals. I found laws inadequate, and public sentiment worse than dead, because of an appetite that had been formed for salacious reading; and especially because decent people could not be made to see or understand the necessity of doing anything in this line. In 1868 Congress had passed a law prohibiting the transmission of obscene books and pictures through the mails. But when in 1872, an effort was made to enforce this law, it was found inadequate. The Legislature of the State of New York had also passed a law, but like the United States law, it only covered a small part of this accursed traffic in human souls.

What was the animus of these men, you ask? I reply, money. Books that sold for $2.50 to $5, cost about 25 cents to make. "But what a business! Who could enjoy money procured in such a manner!" you exclaim. Not so fast, reader. I have arrested over four hundred of these creatures, and every one nearly makes large pretensions to respectability, and say they "must live."

We can acknowledge the daring of the midnight burglar, who creeps into the window of some beautiful home and robs it, or of some highwayman, who, presenting his revolver at the head of his victim, demands "Your money or your life." We can even admit the cunning of the sneak thief, who, watching the thresh-old of the house, creeps in and gathers up his spoil; but how can we find any single saving trait of character in the wretched scoundrel who secretly poisons, debauches and curses the minds of our boys and girls!

It was because of the fatal character and far-reaching extent of this monstrous traffic, and the destruction of young men within my own circle of acquaintances, that I was led, under Providence, in 1872, to undertake the thankless task, so far as it lay in my power, of suppressing this many-sided evil.

I desire to dwell particularly a moment on the history of the Act of Congress of March 3d, 1873, or what the "Liberals" call the "Comstock Law."

This is important on account of the constant cry of the "Liberal" press, that this most important law is "unconstitutional" and "was rushed through without any consideration by the Forty-second Congress."

As the "Liberals" and the writer, in this chapter, are to come directly face to face, we might as well be candid at the start, and talk plainly, and therefore I am very emphatic when I pronounce this claim *maliciously false.*

First. It is malicious, because the United States Supreme Court has, in the case of O. A. Jackson, declared, "that Congress has the right to legislate as to what shall and shall not be carried in the mails," and these men who printed these accusations knew of that decision at the time.

Second. It is false, because there is not a word of truth in it. The facts are, that in the fall or winter of 1872, Hon. Clinton L. Merriam had introduced a bill upon this very subject in the House of Representatives, where he was then a member; again, Hon. Benj. F. Butler of Mass., had introduced another bill on the regulation of commerce between the States; and certain gentleman in Washington had still another bill in the House, all bearing on this very subject.

These measures had all been before the House, and were before the Committees of the House, when I went there in January, 1873. As I have said, the law of 1868 did not meet the requirements of the case. I had prepared a bill, the provisions of which were designed to meet the systemized business which I had found flooding the land through the mails.

The mail of the United States is the great thoroughfare of communication leading up into all our homes, schools and colleges. It is the most powerful agent, to assist this nefarious business, because it *goes everywhere* and *is secret.* It surely needs no argument here to convince the most exacting of all decent men, that no department of Government should be prostituted to serve this infamous traffic, nor become party to it, by continuing to serve these loathsome creatures after the character of their hellish business, with our youth, is known.

When we came to consider the bills that were then before the House of Representatives we found that none of them as drafted, comprehended the wants of the case. Each of the gentlemen and committees were consulted, and all agreed to allow these measures to remain at rest, and give their support to another bill, which was prepared from my rough draft, and which was introduced in the Senate, and referred to the Judiciary Committee.

Then came such an opposition as few bills ever met. "Freedom of the Press is endangered," was the newspaper cry, and they rung the changes on this warning note. One quack in New York, through his clerks, sent to nearly every member of Congress a letter signed by different parties, but all evidently in the same handwriting, calling especial attention to the law, and that it was peculiarly objectionable and ought never to pass; and this letter contained the most infamous libels against myself. I was immediately sent for, and confronted with these base attacks. But when it was found that members of each House had received the same letter from different sources, members examined the bill more carefully. I was called repeatedly before the Committee. I went before large gatherings of Congressmen, and I am positive I personally presented the full facts to a large majority, both in the Senate and House; and after more than a month's consideration, this bill passed the Senate twice unanimously; first on its original passage:

then, after going over to, and passing the House by a minority of but 30, it was sent back with an amendment, and again voted on without a single dissenting voice.

I repeat, this law was *fully* and *carefully examined*, and passed after a *full statement of facts* had been presented.

Down to December, 1877, there had been about three hundred and fifty persons arrested. Many of them had been convicted and sentenced. The quack who sent these base and cowardly letters, had been convicted and sentenced under this law; and something must be done by those whose nefarious business was being so surely broken up. I have been particular about the passage of the law and its uses, because it plays a most interesting and important part in one of the most diabolical schemes to repeal a righteous statute, and ruin a man's good name and reputation by fraud and deception, that has ever come under the writer's attention.

It was really a conspiracy of "smut-dealers;" but as it was operated by a leading so-called "Liberal," and as one hundred and forty out of one hundred and sixty-four Liberal Leagues have arrayed themselves against this work, espousing the cause of the smut-dealer and abortionist, we propose to gratify them by calling the whole movement a LIBERAL FRAUD, and explaining how the "Liberals" manage, when opposing the legal enforcement of righteous laws, and how they endeavored by lying conspiracies, deceit, and fraud, to repeal these laws. At the same time it will illustrate the absolute worthlessness as legislators, of those who advocate no God, no law, no restraining of the libertine and renegade, but a licensing of each individual to follow out his own base designs and purposes.

Surely the blasphemer has found his level; and the adage that "birds of a feather flock together" is proved true.

It is a noted fact, that no sect nor class, as a sect or class, has ever publicly sided with the smut-dealer, and defended this nefarious business, except the Infidels, the Liberals, and the Free-Lovers. The latter are of course in their natural element, and I make no exception for them; but I would be doing violence to the truth and to the golden rule if I did not make some exception to the first two. There are many infidels who abhor this cursed traffic, and several of their papers which for a time were deceived, afterwards came out and openly condemned in strongest terms the acts of these conspirators, and expressed their utter abhorrence of the vile traffic they sought to aid and defend. The same is equally true of many Liberals.

In 1878, the Liberal League while in Convention at Syracuse split on this very subject. The strong, pure, and clean men, those who were honest, and brave enough to stand for moral purity and common decency, under the leadership of Francis E. Abbot, placed themselves emphatically outside the circle of the venders of obscene publications and their sympathizers, by seceding and forming The National Liberal League of America, or what is now known as anti-repealers of obscene publication laws. There were 24 leagues of the strongest men of this fraternity, who left the howling, ranting, blaspheming mob of repealers. For their convictions these men have been ridiculed and maligned by the leaders of these friends of nastiness.

But to return to the fraud.

The basis and motive of this fraud consists, as will be seen, in revenge, avarice, and innate depravity. It possesses not only all the lying and deceit that character-izes these other frauds, but as will also be learned, the conspirators who operated this scheme, sunk to the level of the slanderer and the blackguard, while defend-ing one of the most infamous crimes known to civilization.

While it can hardly be said that this scheme was gotten up for the purpose of enriching these parties who originated it, yet their publications and figures show that they took good care of their own personal interests. Under the thin guise of defending "Freedom of Press," "Free speech," "Free thought," and "Personal Liberty," they entered into a most diabolical conspiracy to repeal the Act of Congress of March 3, 1873, which prohibits obscene publications and articles for indecent and immoral use passing through the mails: and at the same time they sought to crush and ruin the officer who had dared to enforce those laws. In other words, their own nefarious business was endangered because of these righteous laws, and in order to give a decent showing to an indecent and foul busi-ness, they sailed under false colors: and plotted to capture that large class who, believing in no God, are ready to array themselves against anything good and pure. Liberty means license with them, and freedom of press and speech, means that they may, without let or hindrance, blaspheme and deride the holiest things, while any one opposed to their views is to be held to strict accountability. They pay no respect to that very considerable majority, who bow to a Supreme Being, and respect sacred things. These conspirators further sought to show that the proper enforcement of these laws was religious persecution.

The following excerpt comes from the same book. It includes Comstock's interpretation of E. B. Foot's The Book of Nature, *which was excerpted in Appendix A.*

... But next came a PHYSIOLOGICAL STUDENT named E. B. Foote, jr., from the city of New York, the son of a man convicted under these very laws. He was a young man, and if he lives long enough and improves his opportunities, he may learn wisdom. He showed sadly a lack, and also an utter disregard for the truth in what he said before the Committee. He said in substance as follows:

> I am a physiological student. I am hero to represent the physiological side of this subject. This law is no good, there has never been any good accomplished under it. There have been great outrages committed. I know of a reputable physician in the city of New York, who was convicted for sending a purely medical work through the mail. I know the men who are back of this business and who back this man Comstock; they are fanatics and bigots. I am a graduate of one of the medical colleges, and I know

these men well. I have seen their names to papers presented to the Legislature of our State, where I have had occasion to go to have the laws changed that they helped pass.

Others spoke besides these two, and all dealt in the most bitter personalities against me, feeling, doubtless, assured that no person would listen to me after what had been said and done.

At last the suspense is over, the time came for me to speak. I had but one simple duty. Every interest paled before that, *i.e. To show the Committee reasons why the law should not be changed.*

I commenced by calling upon the "physiological student" to witness that what he had said "about no good being done," was untrue; that the first thing accomplished after the signing of the law in 1873 by President Grant, was to oblige his father, Mr. E. B. Foote, of Lexington ave., to suppress several thousands of circulars, advertisements, and books that he was sending through the mails. That the reputable physician who he said had been unjustly convicted for sending "a purely medical work," etc., was his own father, who was convicted not for sending a medical work, but advertisements of an infamous article—an incentive to crime to young girls and women, and that his own clerks testified that the nefarious business was conducted in connection with certain other things they advertised-that the contraband goods were in violation of the laws of the State of New York as well, and that consequently they stored the goods at South Norwalk, Conn., where twice a month a confidential clerk went and filled orders by express; that E. B. Foote received $4.75 out of every $5.00 received through the mails for this infernal article.

Early Motivations for Birth Control—Part II: Feminism, Radicalism, or Public Health?

MARGARET SANGER'S *THE WOMAN REBEL*

Margaret Sanger, *The Woman Rebel: No Gods No Masters*, March 1914, 1, 8, 16.

Margaret Sanger began as a radical advocate for Marxist revolution, which included debunking religious faith and its effect on existing roles for women, expectations of sexual propriety, and the roles of labor and employer. She later narrowed her focus and energies to promoting the cause of legalizing contraception. As a radical, Sanger's voice was limited to a small circle of like-minded friends. But as an advocate of birth control, which was based on her desire for women's safe health, Sanger became a national figure.

A large part of Sanger's success lay in moving the national conversation about birth control away from obscenity (which the public generally opposed) toward new issues of public health (which the public generally supported). Many of her opponents reacted mostly to the radical theories that helped form her support for birth control and ignored the public health side of her arguments. As a result, Sanger began to downplay her previous radicalism and plunged more forcefully into questions of public health, freedom of speech, and religious diversity. By the end of the 1920s, her opponents found themselves without the majority public support that they had previously relied on.

The following selection was taken from Margaret Sanger's first radical newspaper, The Woman Rebel. *This was chosen to stand as a contrast to the Comstock-based temperance ideologies represented in Appendix B. How many of Sanger's presumptions continued throughout the twentieth century? Do any of these presumptions continue to fuel support or opposition to contraception today?*

It will also be the aim of the WOMAN REBEL to advocate the prevention of conception and to impart such knowledge in the columns of this paper.

Other subjects, including the slavery through motherhood; through things, the home, public opinion and so forth, will be dealt with.

It is also the aim of this paper to circulate among those women who work in prostitution; to voice their wrongs; to expose the police persecution which hovers over them and to give free expression to their thoughts, hopes and opinions.

And at all times the WOMAN REBEL will strenuously advocate economic emancipation.

The Prevention of Conception

Is there any reason why women should not receive clean, harmless, scientific knowledge on how to prevent conception? Everybody is aware that the old, stupid fallacy that such knowledge will cause a girl to enter into prostitution has long been shattered. Seldom does a prostitute become pregnant. Seldom does the girl practicing promiscuity become pregnant. The woman of the upper middle class have all available knowledge and implements to prevent conception. The woman of the lower middle class is struggling for this knowledge. She tries various methods of prevention, and after a few years of experience plus medical advice succeeds in discovering some method suitable to her individual self. The woman of the people is the only one left in ignorance of this information. Her neighbors, relatives and friends tell her stories of special devices and the success of them all. They tell her also of the blood-sucking men with M. D. after their names who perform operations for the price of so-and-so. But the working woman's purse is thin. Its far cheaper to have a baby, "though God knows what it will do after it gets here." Then, too, all other classes of women live in places where there is at least a semblance of privacy and sanitation. It is easier for them to care for themselves whereas the large majority of the women of the people have no bathing or sanitary conveniences. This accounts too for the fact that the higher the standard of living, the more care can be taken and fewer children result. No plagues, famine or wars could ever frighten the capitalist class so much as the universal practice of the prevention of conception. On the other hand no better method could be utilized for increasing the wages of the workers.

As is well known, a law exists forbidding the imparting of information on this subject, the penalty being several years' imprisonment. Is it not time to defy this law! And what fitter place could be found than in the pages of the WOMAN REBEL!

Marriage

Marriage, which is a personal agreement between a man and a woman, should be no concern of the State or of the Church. Never have either of these institutions interested themselves in the happiness or health of the individual. Never have they concerned themselves that children be born in healthy and clean surroundings, which might insure their highest development. The Church has been and is anxious only if a child be trained Catholic, Baptist, Methodist and so forth. The State and the Church are concerned only in maintaining and perpetuating themselves even to the detriment and sacrifice of the human race. In the willingness to accept without protest or question the indignities imposed through the barbarities of the Law, together with the stupid superstitions of the Church, can be traced a great proportion of the world's misery.

That there exists in all Nature an attraction which takes place between particles of bodies and unites to form a chemical compound is not doubted. This same attraction exists in men and women and will, unconsciously perhaps, cause them to seek a mate just as other organisms do.

Priests and marriage laws have no power or control over this attraction nor can they make desirable a union where this attraction does not exist.

Marriage laws abrogate the freedom of woman by enforcing upon her a continuous sexual slavery and a compulsory motherhood.

Marriage laws have been dictated and dominated by the Church always and ever upon the unquestionable grounds of the wisdom of the Bible.

A man and woman who under a natural condition avow their love for each other should be immediately qualified by this to give expression to their love or to perpetuate the race without the necessity of a public declaration.

A reciprocal, spontaneous voluntary declaration of love and mutual feelings by a man and woman is the expression of Nature's desires. Were it not natural it would not be so and being natural it is right.

The marriage institution viewed from the light of human experience and the demands of the individual has proven a failure. Statistical reports show that one out of every twelve marriages in the United States has resulted in a divorce—which does not include the thousands of women who want divorces—but on account of the Church and conventions are restrained from obtaining them. Nor does it mention the thousands of women too poor to obtain the price to set in motion the ponderous machinery of the divorce courts. The divorce courts give us only a hint of the dissatisfaction and unhappiness underlying the institution of marriage.

Superstition; blind following; unthinking obedience on the part of working women; together with the pretence, hypocrisy and sham morality of the women of the middle class have been the greatest obstacles in the obtaining of woman's freedom.

Every change in social life is accomplished only by a struggle. Rebel women of the world must fight for the freedom to harmonize their actions with the natural desires of their being, for their deeds are but the concrete expressions of their thoughts.

The Post Office Ban

The woman rebel feels proud the post office authorities did not approve of her. She shall blush with shame if ever she be approved of by officialism of "comstockism."

Rebel Women Wanted

Who deny the right of the State to deprive women of such knowledge as would enable them to take upon themselves voluntary motherhood.

Who deny the right of the State to prohibit such knowledge which would add to the freedom and happiness of the people.

Who demand that those desiring to live together in love shall be provided with such knowledge and experience as Science has developed, which would prevent conception.

Who will assist in the work of increasing the demand for this information.

Who have the courage and backbone to fight with "THE WOMAN REBEL" against this outrageous suppression, whereby a woman has no control of the function of motherhood.

Who are willing to enter this fight, and continue to the end.

Excerpt from *Family Limitation*

Margaret Sanger, *Family Limitation*, 6th ed., 1917.

The following except came from one of Sanger's earlier birth control pamphlets, written with women factory workers in mind. Notice the contrast between the practical instructions of this pamphlet and those used in E. B. Foot's manual.

There is no need for any one to explain to the working men and women in America what this pamphlet is written for or why it is necessary that they should have this information. They know better than I could tell them, so I shall not try.

I have tried to give the knowledge of the best French and Dutch physicians translated into the simplest English, that all may easily understand.

There are various and numerous mechanical means of prevention which I have not mentioned here, mainly because I have not come into personal contact with those who have used them or could recommend them as entirely satisfactory.

I feel there is sufficient information given here, which, if followed, will prevent a woman from becoming pregnant unless she desires to do so.

If a woman is too indolent to wash and cleanse herself, and the man too selfish to consider the consequences of the act, then it will be difficult to find a preventive to keep the woman from becoming pregnant.

Of course, it is troublesome to get up to douche, it is also a nuisance to have to trouble about the date of the menstrual period. It seems inartistic and sordid to insert a pessary or a suppository in anticipation of the sexual act. But it is far more sordid to find yourself several years later burdened down with half a dozen unwanted children, helpless, starved, shoddily clothed, dragging at your skirt, yourself a dragged out shadow of the woman you once were.

Don't be over sentimental in this important phase of hygiene. The inevitable, fact is that unless you prevent the male sperm from entering the womb, you are going to become pregnant. Women of the working class, especially wage workers, should not have more than two children at most. The average working man can support no more and the average working woman can take care of no more in decent fashion. It has been my experience that more children are not really wanted, but that the women are compelled to have them either from lack of foresight or through ignorance of the hygiene of preventing conception.

It is only the workers who are ignorant of the knowledge of how to prevent bringing children in the world to fill jails and hospitals, factories and mills, insane asylums and premature graves.

The working women can use direct action by refusing to supply the market with children to be exploited, by refusing to populate the earth with slaves.

It is also the one most direct method for you working women to help yourself *today*.

Pass on this information to your neighbor and comrade workers. Write out any of the following information which you are sure will help her, and pass it along where it is needed. Spread this important knowledge!

... A Nurse's Advice to Women.

Every woman who is desirous of preventing conception will follow this advice:

Don't wait to see if you do not menstruate (monthly sickness) but make it your duty to see that you *do*.

If you are due to be "sick" on the eighth of August, do not wait until the eighth to see, but begin as early as the fourth to take a good laxative for the bowels, and continue this each night until the eighth.

If there is the slightest possibility that the male fluid has entered the vagina, take on these same nights before retiring, five or ten grains of quinine, with a hot drink. The quinine in capsule form is considered fresher, but if this is taken do not use alcoholic drinks directly after, as it hardens the capsules, thus delaying the action of the quinine.

By taking the above precautions you will prevent the ovum from making its nest in the lining of the womb.

Women of intelligence who refuse to have children until they are ready for them, keep definite track of the date of their menstrual periods. A calendar should be kept, on which can be marked the date of the last menstruation, as well as the date when the next period should occur.

Women must learn to know their own bodies, and watch and know definitely how regular or irregular they are: if the period comes regularly every twenty-eight days (normal) or every thirty days as is in the case of many young girls.

Mark it accordingly on your private calendar; do not leave it to memory or guess work.

Only ignorance and indifference will cause one to be careless in this most important matter.

A very good laxative (though it is a patent medicine) is Beechams Pills. Two of these taken night and morning, four days before menstruation, will give a good cleansing of the bowls and assist with the menstrual flow. Castor oil is also a good laxative.

The American physicians may object to this advice because Beechams Pills are a patent medicine. But until they are willing to give open advice on this subject, we must resort to such as the least harmful, until such time as they do.

If a woman will give herself attention BEFORE the menstrual period arrives, she will almost never have any trouble, but if she neglects herself and waits to see if she "comes around," she is likely to have difficulty.

If the action of quinine has not expelled the semen from the uterus, and a week has elapsed with no signs of the menstrual flow, then it is safe to assume conception has taken place.

Any attempt to interfere with the development of the fertilized ovum is called an abortion.

No one can doubt that there are times where an abortion is justifiable but they will become *unnecessary when care is taken to prevent conception.*

This is the *only* cure for abortions.

. . .

Birth control, or family limitation, has been recommended by some of the leading physicians of the United States and Europe. The movement can no longer be set back by setting up the false cry of "obscenity." It has already been incorporated into the private moral code of millions of the most influential families in every civilized country. It will shortly win full acceptation and sanction by public morality as well.

In cases of women suffering from serious ailments, such as Bright's disease, heart disease, insanities, melancholia, idiocy, consumption, and syphilis, all a physician is allowed to do is to tide these women through their pregnancies if possible. Even though the life of the woman is positively endangered, he cannot relieve her without calling a colleague in consultation. Therefore, the mortality of mothers suffering from these diseases and their infants is very high, and premature births common.

To conserve the lives of these mothers and to prevent the birth of diseased or defective children are factors emphasizing the crying need of a sound and sane educational campaign for birth control.

Excerpts from *What Every Girl Should Know*

Margaret Sanger, *What Every Girl Should Know* (Springfield, IL: United Sales Co., 1920), 90–91.

This selection includes the table of contents, which lists the breadth of information that Sanger believed was necessary for basic sex education. It also includes a selection from the conclusion, which highlights the ideological premises behind Sanger's education agenda.

CHAPTER I: INTRODUCTION
CHAPTER II: GIRLHOOD
    Part 1: Physical Growth
    Part 2: Mental Development
CHAPTER III: PUBERTY
    Part 1: General Organs, Uterus, Ovaries, etc.
    Part 2: Menstruation and Its Disorders
CHAPTER IV: SEXUAL IMPULSE
    Part 1: Masturbation
    Part 2: Sexual Impulse in Animals—in Men—Its Significance in Love
CHAPTER V: REPRODUCTION
    Part 1: Growth of the Life Cell in the Uterus
    Part 2: Hygiene of Pregnancy—Miscarriage
CHAPTER VI: SOME OF THE CONSEQUENCES OF IGNORANCE AND
    SILENCE
    Part 1: Continence in Young Men
    Part 2: Gonorrhea
    Part 3: Syphilis
CHAPTER VII: MENOPAUSE

Conclusion

In conclusion I cannot refrain from saying that women must come to recognize there is some function of womanhood other than being a child-bearing machine. Too long have they allowed themselves to become this, bowing to the yoke of motherhood from puberty to the grave. No other thought has entered the mind except to be a good mother—which has usually meant a slave mother. This has been her only use, her only wish and hope—and when the age arrives where she cannot perform this function longer, she considers herself useless. No wonder she becomes melancholic or even insane.

Fortunately the woman of today is gradually ridding herself of such archaic notions. More and more is she realizing that motherhood is only one of her capabilities; that there are certain individuals more fitted for motherhood than others, just as individuals are better fitted for nursing, teaching, etc.

And further must she realize that though she is past the age of motherhood, yet she is still a woman with all the instincts and experiences which motherhood has bestowed upon her, and she can now begin a new development, based upon these valuable experiences, she can now enter into public life unhampered by the details of kitchen and babies, for as she completes her work and passes on, others come in to take her place.

Being free from domestic and maternal cares enables her to give to society the benefit of her matured thought, seasoned and enriched by these experiences.

She often does enjoy the best health of her life after the Menopause and this, together with a vista of a future of usefulness, should open to the woman in the post-climateric period, a new life—a new world.

In completing this series of articles I cannot refrain from uttering just a word about the relation of the entire subject I have been discussing to the economic problem. It is impossible to separate the ignorance of parents, prostitution, venereal diseases, or the silence of the medical profession from the great economic questions that the world is facing today. It is here ever before us, and the more we look into the so-called evils of the day the more we realize that the whole structure of the present day society is built upon a rotten and decaying foundation. Until capitalism is swept away, there is no hope for young girls to live a beautiful life during their girlhood. There is no hope for boys or girls to build up strong and sturdy bodies. There is no hope that a woman can live in the family relation and have children without sacrificing every vestige of individual development. There is no hope that prostitution will cease, as long as there is hunger. There is no hope for a strong race as long as venereal diseases exist. And they will exist until women rise in one big sisterhood to fight this capitalist society which compels a woman to serve as a sex implement for man's use.

Education is necessary—education is the need of the people. For this will soon enable one to see that knowledge alone does not suffice, but that it is only through economic security that the man and the woman will emerge in a future civilization.

EXCERPT FROM THE SANGER-RUSSELL DEBATE ON BIRTH CONTROL

E. Haldeman-Julius, *Debate on Birth Control: Mrs. Sanger and W. Russell and Shaw vs. Roosevelt on Birth Control* (Girard, KS: Haldeman-Julius Company, 1921), 4–9, 44–45, 47 (Winter); 9–11, 13–14, 15–17, 20–21, 40.

Margaret Sanger engaged in a number of debates on the issue of birth control and published some of them later. This selection is from a debate published through Sanger's organization, so it does not necessarily provide the best example of Sanger's opponents. Nevertheless, the exchange reveals some of the arguments that motivated both sides of the issue in the early 1920s. Some of these arguments remain relevant for modern discussions. Of particular interest is the continuation of temperance-based arguments on the opposition side and the new public health arguments presented on the proponent side. Notice also how some of the other points, both for and against contraception, would no longer be welcome on either side of modern debates.

Winter Russell—First Speech

Mr. Russell: We are going to deal with these principles. I am not going to concern myself much with authorities. I suppose she can quote from Dr. Robinson and apparently Dr. Knopf (he says he isn't an authority,) and others as authorities. I could quote from Lamb and Roosevelt and the Bible—the great religions of the earth—scriptural authority that comes from the very depths of the spiritual, and what I believe to be the very mouth of God itself—of Nature—If you do not like to admit the existence of Providence.

I am not concerned with Scripture or authorities. I am going to deal with this question from what I believe are the cold, inevitable facts of life as we know them, and meet them every day.

Now I am going to admit in the first place that there are many families with too many children. It would be foolish to gainsay that. They are a burden to the mother. They are a hardship to the father who tries to provide for them. They make conditions unfair and unjust for the other children. The fact is, and I hope that she will admit it also, that there are thousands of homes in the United States of America that are too lacking In children—although I think she has once stated that the most immoral thing a person can do is to bring a large family into the world. Here we have the problem and the question is, how are we going to meet it?

I propose that we should meet this problem by the measure of self-control. I believe by this means we can solve it, and at the same time gain one of the greatest advantages you can possibly win on the face of the earth. Sex control is the best path to self-control and to self-discipline. It is the key to wisdom. It is the key to power. It is the key to intellectual and mental development; indeed, she has once stated that only those people who are mentally developed are capable of self-control and I want to say that they got a large measure of their mental development by self-control. She is looking through the wrong end of the telescope.

And so we come to this method. I want to say, as another part of the platform upon which I am to stand, that I conceive and hold marriage to be more than physical. It is not a purely sensual relationship. It borders on the aesthetic, spiritual, mental, and modern aspects of life, and when you try to take the physical by itself you find a condition of naked sensuality which is disastrous in the extreme.

My contentions are these: In the first place, fundamentally, universally, infinitely from every point of view, [naked sensuality] is vicious. It is false from every scientific construction that you can possibly conceive of; it is one of the most vitiating things from every point of philosophy, physiology and psychology.

I believe [birth control] is disastrous intellectually, mentally, and spiritually. It is disastrous and perpetrates a great wrong upon the unborn millions who are waiting for entrance upon this great amphitheatre of life. It is disastrous physically, mentally, and spiritually upon the future. It is disastrous to the same degree upon the people who practice it—husbands and wives who resort to these measures. I hold that it perpetrates the greatest crime of all the ages, namely, race suicide.

Let us approach the first method, and that is this question of whether it is right from the point of view of the philosophy of man, if you will; and I want you to consider it simply from the practical living point of view. I want to lay down this proposition—it is that you can't have pleasure in this world without paying for it—that there are certain laws that sweep through the entire universe from the furthest star to the tiniest atom and molecule that you can find in existence.

I am a member of the bar or the State of New York. I trust that I have due regard and respect for the statutes, the constitution and the laws or this great city, state and nation. But I hold them as the veriest trash when they come up against the laws of Nature. The laws of Nature cannot be revised. They cannot be repealed. There is no power in this whole universe that can change these laws with which you have to deal.

That means you can't get pleasure without paying for it. Nature is inexorable in bringing about her retribution. She does not need any balance book. You can never embezzle. You can't cheat. You can't get away from her.

Emerson has said that "the ingenuity of man has always been dedicated to the solution of one problem—how to detach the sensual sweet, the sensual strong, the sensual bright from the moral sweet, the moral deep, the moral fair—that is again to contrive to cut clean off this upper surface so thin as to leave it bottomless, to get one end without the other end. The soul says eat, the body would feast. The soul says, 'The man and woman shall be one flesh and one soul.' The body would join the flesh only."

"All things are double, one against the other," continued Emerson. "Tit for tat. An eye for an eye, tooth for a tooth, blood for blood, measure for measure, love for love. Give and it shall be given you. He that watereth shall be watered himself. What will you have, quoth God, pay for it and take it. Nothing ventured, nothing have. Thou shalt be paid exactly for what thou has done, no more, no less. Who doth not work, doth not eat. Harm watch, harm catch. Curses always recoil on the head of him who imprecates them. If you chain a slave, one end chains you. Bad counsel confounds the adviser. The devil is an ass."

You must pay at last your own debt. Those are the laws. Now we recognize it in physics. Energy cannot be annihilated. Birth control says, "yes." You shall pay the price. You can annihilate that energy and drink from the cup of pleasure, but you don't take the responsibility—the duty and the care. You recognize it in physics. You recognize it in chemistry, in every law of life. When Ponzi in Boston said, "I will give you 50 percent"—the world laughed, because it can't be done. Birth control advocates, like the Ponzis, say they will give you 50 percent and 100 percent on your investment, but it can't be done. It is frenzied finance. It is along the lines of the people who are alchemists, who think they can turn the baser metals into gold. It is an age-long dream. It is a belief that has been held from the beginning of time. That thing cannot be done. That is the law of life— of God—that you have to pay.

And so that is the thing you are confronted with. I don't say that you don't seem to gain, but for every gain you seem to grasp you have lost the life of it. He who does not work shall not eat. The trouble is that we are bound by the fetish of money, of gold, and lose sight. In other words we have eyes literally that see not, and ears that hear not.

And that is the thing that we must consider. So I want you to have in mind, that by the very law of life, the very theory of science of our being, we have to pay, and if we take that, if we try to grasp that, we are going to pay the penalty. In my next opportunity to address you I shall take up that to show you how we pay. (Applause.)

... As I look at America today, I see it in the grip of a foul monster. It was as though we had been gassed. I consider these teachings as mental and spiritual dope. Morphine and heroin don't compare with the way in which we are duped today. It speaks in all of our literature and customs. When you see a woman in a pregnant condition today, you see smirks and snubs as though it was a misfortune to that poor woman.

Take the intellectual life of America today. Greenwich Village thinks it is intellectual. It is the intellectual sewage disposal plant of America today, and it is not very scientific. It is a fact. Fifth Avenue and the west side where I live—it is the social garbage dumping grounds of the Nation. All these people want is freedom and liberty—freedom to be foul, freedom and liberty—freedom to be foul, freedom to be disgusting—they think they can obtain pleasure without paying for it. If there is anything that annoys me and my nerves is this puking pus that is called love poured forth over the poodle dog by volunteer married person today.

As a matter of fact, a large family is the hope of the world. It is the greatest disciplinary force that there is in life. That is nothing that so develops the mind and soul of a man and woman as bringing up a great family of children. These disciplinary forces we are losing today and that is because we are following the easiest way. We are taking the course of the least resistance. You are trying to get the honey and escape the thorns, and it can't be done.

... I believe that the great mass of so-called Americans are today voluntarily but blindly shutting the unborn out from the Heaven to which I hope we will all ultimately reach.

Margaret Sanger—First Speech

Mrs. Sanger: Mr. Chairman, and ladies and gentlemen. Mr. Russell and I seem to agree on some of the points of this argument, at least, but as usual with most opponents of birth control, they have absolutely no intelligent argument. (Laughter.) They always barricade themselves behind the Bible or the terrible vengeance of an offended Nature. That is exactly what Mr. Russell is doing now.

Now, friends, I want to say, let us get down to fundamental principles. Let us get together and look at life the way it is now, not as it might have been had

Nature acted thus and so, not as it might be had God done thus and so, but as we find ourselves today. We have a few principles of life by which we must live, and I claim that everyone of us has a right to health, to liberty and to the pursuit of happiness. I say furthermore that birth control is an absolutely essential factor in our living and having those three principles of happiness. (Applause.)

By birth control, I mean a voluntary, conscious control of the birth rate by means that prevent conception—scientific means that prevent conception. I don't mean birth control by abstinence or by continence or anything except the thing that agrees with most of us, and as we will develop later on, most of are glad that there are means of science at the present time that are not injurious, not harmful, and all conception can be avoided.

Now let us look upon life as it really is, and we see society today is divided distinctly into two groups: those who use the means of birth control and those who do not.

On the one side we find those who do use means in controlling birth. What have they? They are the people who bring to birth few children. They are the people who have all the happiness, who have wealth and the leisure for culture and mental and spiritual development. They are people who rear their children to manhood and womanhood and who fill the universities and the colleges with their progeny. Nature has seemed to be very kind to that group of people. (Laughter.)

On the other hand we have the group who have large families and have for generations perpetuated large families, and I know from work among them that the great percentage of these people that are brought into the world in poverty and misery have been unwanted, I know that most of these women are just as desirous to have means to control birth as the women of wealth. I know she tries desperately to obtain the information, not for selfish purposes, but for her own benefit and for that of her children. In this group, what we have? We have poverty, misery, disease, overcrowding, congestion, child labor, infant mortality, maternal mortality, all the evils which today are grouped in the crowd where there are large families of unwanted and undesired children.

Take the first one and let us see how these mothers feel. I claim that a woman, whether she is rich or poor, has a right to be a mother or not when she feels herself fit to be so. She has just as much right not to be a mother as she has to be a mother. It is just as right and as moral for people to talk of small families and to demand them as to want large families. It is just as moral.

... The only weapon that women have, and the most uncivilized weapon that they must use, if they will not submit to having children every year and a half, is abortion. We know how detrimental abortion is to the physical side as well as to the psychic side of woman's life. Yet there are in this nation, because of these generalities and opinions that are here before us, and that are stopping the tide of progress, more than one million women who have abortions performed on them each year.

What does this mean? It is a very bad sign when women indulge in it, and it means they are absolutely determined that they cannot continue bringing children into the world that they cannot clothe, feed and shelter. It is a woman's instinct, and she knows herself when she should and should not give birth to children, and it is much more natural to trust this instinct and to let her be the judge than it is to let her judge herself by some unknown God. I claim it is a woman's duty and right to have for herself the power to say when she shall and shall not have children.

. . . We speak of the rights of the unborn. I say that it is time to speak for those who are already born. I also say and know that the infant death rate is affected tremendously by those who arrive last. The first child that comes—the first or second or third child which arrives in a family, has a far better chance than those that arrive later.

. . . We know that the mothers and fathers of today produce the race of tomorrow, and we know that unless we have a clean child and a clean stream of blood flowing through that child that the race of tomorrow is a doomed and foregone conclusion. We know, too, that out of this terrible scourge of disease comes 90 percent of the insanity in this country, due to syphilis. Anyone who is dealing with fundamentals would know that these people should use means to protect themselves against having children. They should absolutely, in due regard to themselves, to their children and to the race, not allow a child to be born while that disease is running riot in the system. The terrible consequence is insanity.

. . . Now we look upon all these things in just about the same way. We try to palliate most all of them. Take one instance—our immigration laws. The United States Government makes the most rigid laws. It scans the vessels carefully to see that no one should enter who is an idiot, who is insane, and who is a pauper. They see to it that anyone who enters is not an idiot, is not insane and is not a pauper. They make those rigid laws and rules for those who shall come in, but after you are once on the inside, you can produce and reproduce and repopulate the earth with syphilitic and diseased and insane people so far as the government is concerned. This is the shortsighted side of our whole life. We are very generous and sympathetic but we are over sentimental and the time has come to use our minds and to apply our intelligence to life and to the conditions of life as we find them today.

. . . Birth control is the pivot around which every movement must swing making for race betterment. Birth control does not act as a substitute for any social scheme or other ideal system. But it must be the base and serve them as a foundation.

Birth control will free the mother from the trap of pregnancy. It will save the child from that procession of coffins, as well as from the toil of mill and factory.

Birth control will make parenthood a voluntary function instead of an accident as it is today. When motherhood and childhood are free, we then can go hand in hand toward the emancipation of the human race.

Supreme Court Cases—From Public Health to Civil Rights

Moral arguments may be the most enduring deeply rooted cause for opposition to contraception, but such arguments have less meaning in our increasingly pluralistic society. Throughout the 1950s and 1960s, the Supreme Court debated whether it had an obligation to interpret rights that were not explicitly stipulated in the Constitution. Among these was the "right to privacy," which grew out of the 1965 decision of Griswold v. Connecticut, *which ruled that the Connecticut law outlawing the sale and distribution of contraceptives was unconstitutional. This decision became the basis for the later controversial decision of* Roe v. Wade, *which applied the same right to privacy to state laws prohibiting abortion. The effective consequence of these rulings was to remove matters of public morality as a relevant consideration for state lawmakers. The churches may debate the morality of artificial contraceptives, but jurists and lawmakers no longer will.*

Since it is currently less feasible to use moral positions to challenge public policy, critics are forced to use other reasons that have greater legal bearing, such as "voluntariness" and "consumer protection." Nevertheless, the practical reality is that most opposition to birth control still stems from deeply held moral positions.

These selections were chosen to demonstrate the trend of the Supreme Court in its decisions over contraception in the twentieth century. In the early decades, the Court accepted the state's right to legislate matters of sterilization and contraception for the sake of public morality and public health. By the end of the century, the Court was arguing the exact opposite.

Excerpt from *Buck v. Bell*

Buck v. Bell, 274 U.S. 200 (1927); argued April 22, 1927; decided May 2, 1927.

Prior to the 1950s, the U.S.Supreme Court rarely interfered with criminal codes passed by individual state legislatures. When they did consider such cases, frequently the Court chose not to interfere unless the state law explicitly violated specific provisions in the U.S. Constitution. On matters that bridged criminal codes and public morality, the Court remained even more restrained. Between 1900 and the 1930s, many states passed laws that prescribed involuntary sterilization for certain types of criminals and for those judged "insane" or "feebleminded." When the constitutionality of these laws reached the Court in Buck v. Bell *in 1927, the Court chose not to interfere and upheld the state's right to regulate reproduction for the sake of public health.*

Compare the arguments in this case to those made in Griswold v. Connecticut *to see the extent to which the Supreme Court changed its approach. Justice Holmes clearly relied on eugenics arguments to base his decision. Although such arguments were no longer viable after World War II, many other issues from* Buck v. Bell *continue to influence debates of public support for birth control: When does a public funded family planning program cease to be voluntary? Do the needs of public health trump individual rights? Should states provide contraceptives to minors without parental consent?*

Mr. JUSTICE HOLMES delivered the opinion of the Court

This is a writ of error to review a judgment of the Supreme Court of Appeals of the State of Virginia affirming a judgment of the Circuit Court of Amherst County by which the defendant in error, the superintendent of the State Colony for Epileptics and Feeble Minded, was ordered to perform the operation of salpingectomy upon Carrie Buck, the plaintiff in error, for the purpose of making her sterile. . . . The case comes here upon the contention that the statute authorizing the judgment is void under the Fourteenth Amendment as denying to the plaintiff in error due process of law and the equal protection of the laws.

Carrie Buck is a feeble minded white woman who was committed to [Virginia State Colony for Epileptics and Feeble Minded] in due form. She is the daughter of a feeble minded mother in the same institution, and the mother of an illegitimate feeble minded child. She was eighteen years old at the time of the trial of her case in the Circuit Court, in the latter part of 1924. An Act of Virginia, approved March 20, 1924, recites that the health of the patient and the welfare of society may be promoted in certain cases by the sterilization of mental defectives, under careful safeguard, &c.; that the sterilization may be effected in males by vasectomy and in females by salpingectomy, without serious pain or substantial danger to life; that the Commonwealth is supporting in various institutions many defective persons who, if now discharged, would become a menace, but, if incapable of procreating, might be discharged with safety and become self-supporting with benefit to themselves and to society, and that experience has shown that heredity plays an important part in the transmission of insanity, imbecility, & c. The statute then enacts that, whenever the superintendent of certain institutions, including the above-named State Colony, shall be of opinion that it is for the best interests of the patients and of society that an inmate under his care should be sexually sterilized, he may have the operation performed upon any patient afflicted with hereditary forms of insanity, imbecility, &c., on complying with the very careful provisions by which the act protects the patients from possible abuse.

The superintendent first presents a petition to the special board of directors of his hospital or colony, stating the facts and the grounds for his opinion, verified by affidavit. Notice of the petition and of the time and place of the hearing in the institution is to be served upon the inmate, and also upon his guardian, and if there is no guardian, the superintendent is to apply to the Circuit Court of the County to appoint one. If the inmate is a minor, notice also is to be given to his parents, if any, with a copy of the petition. The board is to see to it that the inmate may attend the hearings if desired by him or his guardian. The evidence is all to be reduced to writing, and, after the board has made its order for or against the operation, the superintendent, or the inmate, or his guardian, may appeal to the Circuit Court of the County. The Circuit Court may consider the record of the board and the evidence before it and such other admissible evidence as may be offered, and may affirm, revise, or reverse the order of the board and enter such order as it deems just. Finally any party may apply to the Supreme Court of Appeals, which, if it grants the appeal, is to hear the case upon the record of the trial in the Circuit Court, and may enter such order as it thinks the Circuit Court should have entered. There can be no doubt that, so far as procedure is concerned, the rights of the patient are most carefully considered, and, as every step in this case was taken in scrupulous compliance with the statute and after months of observation, there is no doubt that, in that respect, the plaintiff in error has had due process of law.

The attack is not upon the procedure, but upon the substantive law. It seems to be contended that in no circumstances could such an order be justified. It certainly is contended that the order cannot be justified upon the existing grounds. The judgment finds the facts that have been recited, and that Carrie Buck "is the probable potential parent of socially inadequate offspring, likewise afflicted, that she may be sexually sterilized without detriment to her general health, and that her welfare and that of society will be promoted by her sterilization," and thereupon makes the order. In view of the general declarations of the legislature and the specific findings of the Court, obviously we cannot say as matter of law that the grounds do not exist, and, if they exist, they justify the result. We have seen more than once that the public welfare may call upon the best citizens for their lives. It would be strange if it could not call upon those who already sap the strength of the State for these lesser sacrifices, often not felt to be such by those concerned, in order to prevent our being swamped with incompetence. It is better for all the world if, instead of waiting to execute degenerate offspring for crime or to let them starve for their imbecility, society can prevent those who are manifestly unfit from continuing their kind. The principle that sustains compulsory vaccination is broad enough to cover cutting the Fallopian tubes. . . . Three generations of imbeciles are enough.

But, it is said, however it might be if this reasoning were applied generally, it fails when it is confined to the small number who are in the institutions named and is not applied to the multitudes outside. It is the usual last resort of constitutional arguments to point out shortcomings of this sort. But the answer is that the law does all that is needed when it does all that it can, indicates a policy, applies it to all within the lines, and seeks to bring within the lines all similarly situated so far and so fast as its means allow. Of course, so far as the operations enable those who otherwise must be kept confined to be returned to the world, and thus open the asylum to others, the equality aimed at will be more nearly reached.

Judgment affirmed.

EXCERPT FROM *UNITED STATES V. ONE PACKAGE*

United States v. One Package, No. 62, Circuit Court of Appeals, Second Circuit, 86 F.2d 737; 1936 U.S. App. LEXIS 3844, December 7, 1936.

Less than 10 years after Buck v. Bell, *the Second Circuit Court of Appeals heard a case challenging one of the state-based Comstock laws that prohibited contraceptives from being sent through the mails. Notice that the appellate court does not deny the state's right to safeguard the morality of the public. Instead, it focuses only on doctors' rights to prescribe necessary remedies, including contraceptives, if doctors believe that health risks are at stake. In this instance, the appellate court views the needs of public health to be more important than the state's right to protect public immorality.*

This case paved the way legalizing any and all research related to contraception while also allowing virtually any doctor in any state to prescribe contraceptives at will. It did not, however, deny the state's right to protect public morality by limiting or banning contraceptives for the general public.

Augustus N. Hand, Circuit Judge

The claimant Dr. Stone is a New York physician who has been licensed to practice for sixteen years and has specialized in gynecology. The package containing [120 vaginal pessaries] was sent to her by a physician in Japan for the purpose of trying them in her practice and giving her opinion as to their usefulness for contraceptive purposes. She testified that she prescribes the use of pessaries in cases where it would not be desirable for a patient to undertake a pregnancy. The accuracy and good faith of this testimony is not questioned. The New York Penal Law, which makes it in general a misdemeanor to sell or give away or to advertise or offer for sale any articles for the prevention of conception, excepts furnishing such articles to physicians who may in good faith prescribe their use for the cure or prevention of disease. . . . The witnesses for both the government and the claimant testified that the use of contraceptives was in many cases necessary for the health of women and that they employed articles of the general nature of the pessaries in their practice. There was no dispute as to the truth of these statements.

The question is whether physicians who import such articles as those involved in the present case in order to use them for the health of their patients are excepted by implication from the literal terms of the statute. Certainly they are excepted in the case of an abortive which is prescribed to save life, for section 305(a) of the Tariff Act only prohibits the importation of articles for causing "unlawful abortion." This was the very point decided in *Bours v. United States*, . . . where a similar statute . . . declaring nonmailable "every article or thing designed, adapted, or intended for preventing conception or producing abortion, or for any indecent or immoral use," was held not to cover physicians using the mails in order to say that they will operate upon a patient if an examination shows the necessity of an operation to save life. And this result was reached even though the statute in forbidding the mailing of any article "intended for . . . producing abortion" did not, as does section 305(a) of the Tariff Act, qualify the word "abortion" by the saving adjective "unlawful."

. . . Section 305(a) of the Tariff Act of 1930, as well as title 18, section 334, of the U.S. Code . . . prohibiting the mailing, and title 18, section 396 of the U.S. Code, . . . prohibiting the importing or transporting in interstate commerce of articles "designed, adapted, or intended for preventing conception, or producing abortion," all originated from the so-called Comstock Act of 1873, . . . which was entitled "An Act for the Suppression of Trade in, and Circulation of, obscene Literature and Articles of immoral Use."

Section 1 of the act of 1873 made it a crime to sell, lend, or give away, "any drug or medicine, or any article whatever, for the prevention of conception, or for causing unlawful abortion." Section 2 prohibited sending through the mails "any article or thing designed or intended for the prevention of conception or procuring of abortion." Section 3 forbade the importation of "any of the hereinbefore-mentioned articles or things, except the drugs here in beforementioned when imported in bulk, and not put up for any of the purposes before mentioned." All the statutes we have referred to were part of a continuous scheme to suppress immoral articles and obscene literature and should so far as possible be construed together and consistently. If this be done, the articles here in question ought not to be forfeited when not intended for an immoral purpose . . .

It is true that in 1873, when the Comstock Act was passed, information now available as to the evils resulting in many cases from conception was most limited, and accordingly it is argued that the language prohibiting the sale or mailing of contraceptives should be taken literally and that Congress intended to bar the use of such articles completely. While we may assume that section 305(a) of the Tariff Act of 1930 . . . exempts only such articles as the act of 1873 excepted, yet we are satisfied that this statute, as well as all the acts we have referred to, embraced only such articles as Congress would have denounced as immoral if it had understood all the conditions under which they were to be used. Its design, in our opinion, was not to prevent the importation, sale, or carriage by mail of things which might intelligently be employed by conscientious and competent physicians for the purpose of saving life or promoting the well being of their patients.... While it is true that the policy of Congress has been to forbid the use of contraceptives altogether if the only purpose of using them be to prevent conception in cases where it would not be injurious to the welfare of the patient or her offspring, it is going far beyond such a policy to hold that abortions, which destroy incipient life, may be allowed in proper cases, and yet that no measures may be taken to prevent conception even though a likely result should be to require the termination of pregnancy by means of an operation. It seems unreasonable to suppose that the national scheme of legislation involves such inconsistencies and requires the complete suppression of articles, the use of which in many cases is advocated by such a weight of authority in the medical world.

The Comstock Bill, as originally introduced in the Senate, contained the words "except on a prescription of a physician in good standing, given in good faith," but those words were omitted from the bill as it was ultimately passed. The reason for amendment seems never to have been discussed on the floor of Congress, or in committee, and the remarks of Senator Conklin, when the bill was up for passage in final form, indicate that the scope of the measure was not well understood and that the language used was to be left largely for future interpretation. We see no ground for holding that the construction placed upon similar language in the decisions we have referred to is not applicable to the articles which the government seeks to forfeit, and common sense would seem to require a like interpretation in the case at bar.

The decree dismissing the libel is affirmed.

L. Hand, Circuit Judge (Concurring)

If the decision had been left to me alone, I should have felt more strongly than my brothers the force of the Senate amendment in the original act, and of the use of the word, "unlawful," as it passed. There seems to me substantial reason for saying that contraconceptives were meant to be forbidden, whether or not prescribed by physicians, and that no lawful use of them was contemplated. Many people have changed their minds about such matters in sixty years, but the act forbids the same conduct now as then; a statute stands until public feeling gets enough momentum to change it, which may be long after a majority would repeal it, if a poll were taken. Nevertheless, I am not prepared to dissent. I recognize that the course of the act through Congress does not tell us very much, and it is of considerable importance that the law as to importations should be the same as that as to the mails; we ought not impute differences of intention upon slight distinctions in expression. I am content therefore to accept my brothers' judgment, whatever might have been, and indeed still are, my doubts.

Excerpt from *Griswold v. Connecticut*

Griswold et al. v. Connecticut, 381 U.S. 479; 85 S. Ct. 1678; 14 L. Ed. 2d 510; 1965 U.S. LEXIS 2282.

During the 1950s, the Supreme Court under Chief Justice Earl Warren passed a number of decisions that led to dramatic social changes in the area of civil rights, including desegregation of schools, housing, and eventually all public facilities at the state levels. Following on these decisions, the Court then moved into the field of criminals codes, which, with few exceptions, are based on state laws. Armed with the goal of protecting the rights of the accused (whether guilty or not), the Warren Court issued a series of landmark decisions resulting in a host of federal regulations over criminal due process. It was in this period that the Court chose to take up the question of whether states could outlaw the use of contraceptives.

Since no state had enforced its "Comstock laws" in more than 50 years, most of the discussion relevant to this case dealt with theoretical powers of the Court to oversee state laws. Griswold v. Connecticut *stands as a landmark case because it launched a new constitutional construct called the "right to privacy." It later served as the basis for a number of other cases, including the controversial* Roe v. Wade, *which was decided eight years later.*

Griswold was decided by a slim five-to-four majority, but what is more revealing is that no more than three justices agreed on why they supported (or opposed) the final decision. In this way, Griswold *provides a remarkable look into some of the most critical constitutional debates of the twentieth century. Attention should be paid to the three separate explanations for why the Connecticut law should be overturned——note that they are not necessarily compatible with each other. One interpretation relies on broad interpretations of specific amendments, while another introduces a novel interpretation of the Ninth Amendment, and the last asserts that no specific amendment is necessary to overturn a state law that violates "natural justice." The dissenting views criticize each of the three variations for inventing constitutional rights that do not exist.*

A highly charged political debate continues over whether judges should adopt a strict construction of the Constitution or whether they should adopt a more flexible interpretation to better adapt the document to the "changing times" and is a major dividing point between Republicans and Democrats. The fact that both contraceptives and abortion helped to frame this constitutional debate almost guarantees that each new policy involving either contraception or abortion will involve political controversy. For the most part, abortion-related policies are more polarizing, but a similar strain of resistance also follows public funding of contraceptives. Although moral questions fuel most of the criticism against artificial methods of birth control, there is also another source of criticism based on political ideologies that opposed the process by which contraceptives and abortion were legalized.

MR. JUSTICE DOUGLAS delivered the opinion of the Court

Appellant Griswold is Executive Director of the Planned Parenthood League of Connecticut. Appellant Buxton is a licensed physician and a professor at the Yale Medical School who served as Medical Director for the League at its Center in New Haven—a center open and operating from November 1 to November 10, 1961, when appellants were arrested.

They gave information, instruction, and medical advice to married persons as to the means of preventing conception. They examined the wife and prescribed the best contraceptive device or material for her use. Fees were usually charged, although some couples were serviced free.

The statutes whose constitutionality is involved in this appeal are §§ 53-32 and 54-196 of the General Statutes of Connecticut (1958 rev.). The former provides:

Any person who uses any drug, medicinal article or instrument for the purpose of preventing conception shall be fined not less than fifty dollars or imprisoned not less than sixty days nor more than one year or be both fined and imprisoned.

Section 54-196 provides:

Any person who assists, abets, counsels, causes, hires or commands another to commit any offense may be prosecuted and punished as if he were the principal offender.

The appellants were found guilty as accessories and fined $100 each, against the claim that the accessory statute as so applied violated the Fourteenth Amendment. The Appellate Division of the Circuit Court affirmed. The Supreme Court of Errors affirmed that judgment

. . .

Coming to the merits, we are met with a wide range of questions that implicate the Due Process Clause of the Fourteenth Amendment. Overtones of some arguments suggest that *Lochner v. New York*, . . . should be our guide. But we decline that invitation as we did in [other cases]. . . . We do not sit as a super-legislature to determine the wisdom, need, and propriety of laws that touch economic problems, business affairs, or social conditions. This law, however, operates directly on an intimate relation of husband and wife and their physician's role in one aspect of that relation.

The association of people is not mentioned in the Constitution nor in the Bill of Rights. The right to educate a child in a school of the parents' choice—whether public or private or parochial—is also not mentioned. Nor is the right to study any particular subject or any foreign language. Yet the First Amendment has been construed to include certain of those rights . . .

In other words, the State may not, consistently with the spirit of the First Amendment, contract the spectrum of available knowledge. The right of freedom of speech and press includes not only the right to utter or to print, but the right to distribute, the right to receive, the right to read . . . and freedom of inquiry, freedom of thought, and freedom to teach . . . —indeed the freedom of the entire university community. . . . Without those peripheral rights the specific rights would be less secure . . .

[T]he First Amendment has a penumbra where privacy is protected from governmental intrusion. In like context, we have protected forms of "association" that are not political in the customary sense but pertain to the social, legal, and economic benefit of the members. . . . The right of "association," like the right of belief . . . is more than the right to attend a meeting; it includes the right to express one's attitudes or philosophies by membership in a group or by affiliation with it or by other lawful means. Association in that context is a form of expression of opinion; and while it is not expressly included in the First Amendment its existence is necessary in making the express guarantees fully meaningful.

The foregoing cases suggest that specific guarantees in the Bill of Rights have penumbras, formed by emanations from those guarantees that help give them life and substance. . . . Various guarantees create zones of privacy. The right of association contained in the penumbra of the First Amendment is one, as we have seen. The Third Amendment in its prohibition against the quartering of soldiers "in any house" in time of peace without the consent of the owner is another facet of that privacy. The Fourth Amendment explicitly affirms the "right of the people to be secure in their persons, houses, papers, and effects, against unreasonable searches and seizures." The Fifth Amendment in its Self-Incrimination Clause enables the citizen to create a zone of privacy which government may not force him to surrender to his detriment. The Ninth Amendment provides: "The enumeration in the Constitution, of certain rights, shall not be construed to deny or disparage others retained by the people."

. . . The present case, then, concerns a relationship lying within the zone of privacy created by several fundamental constitutional guarantees. And it concerns a law which, in forbidding the use of contraceptives rather than regulating their manufacture or sale, seeks to achieve its goals by means having a maximum destructive impact upon that relationship. Such a law cannot stand in light of the familiar principle, so often applied by this Court, that a "governmental purpose to control or prevent activities constitutionally subject to state regulation may not be achieved by means which sweep unnecessarily broadly and thereby invade the area of protected freedoms." *NAACP v. Alabama*. . . . Would we allow the police to search the sacred precincts of marital bedrooms for telltale signs of the use of contraceptives? The very idea is repulsive to the notions of privacy surrounding the marriage relationship.

We deal with a right of privacy older than the Bill of Rights—older than our political parties, older than our school system. Marriage is a coming together for better or for worse, hopefully enduring, and intimate to the degree of being sacred. It is an association that promotes a way of life, not causes; a harmony in living, not political faiths; a bilateral loyalty, not commercial or social projects. Yet it is an association for as noble a purpose as any involved in our prior decisions.

Reversed . . .

MR. JUSTICE GOLDBERG, whom THE CHIEF JUSTICE and MR. JUSTICE BRENNAN join, concurring

I agree with the Court that Connecticut's birth-control law unconstitutionally intrudes upon the right of marital privacy, and I join in its opinion and judgment. Although I have not accepted the view that "due process" as used in the Fourteenth Amendment incorporates all of the first eight Amendments ... I do agree that the concept of liberty protects those personal rights that are fundamental, and is not confined to the specific terms of the Bill of Rights. My conclusion that the concept of liberty is not so restricted and that it embraces the right of marital privacy though that right is not mentioned explicitly in the Constitution is supported both by numerous decisions of this Court, referred to in the Court's opinion, and by the language and history of the Ninth Amendment ...

In determining which rights are fundamental, judges are not left at large to decide cases in light of their personal and private notions. Rather, they must look to the "traditions and [collective] conscience of our people" to determine whether a principle is "so rooted [there] ... as to be ranked as fundamental." *Snyder v. Massachusetts* ... The inquiry is whether a right involved "is of such a character that it cannot be denied without violating those 'fundamental principles of liberty and justice which lie at the base of all our civil and political institutions'" ... *Powell v. Alabama*. ... "Liberty" also "gains content from the emanations of ... specific [constitutional] guarantees" and "from experience with the requirements of a free society." *Poe v. Ullman*. ...

I agree fully with the Court that, applying these tests, the right of privacy is a fundamental personal right, emanating "from the totality of the constitutional scheme under which we live." ...

The entire fabric of the Constitution and the purposes that clearly underlie its specific guarantees demonstrate that the rights to marital privacy and to marry and raise a family are of similar order and magnitude as the fundamental rights specifically protected.

Although the Constitution does not speak in so many words of the right of privacy in marriage, I cannot believe that it offers these fundamental rights no protection. The fact that no particular provision of the Constitution explicitly forbids the State from disrupting the traditional relation of the family—a relation as old and as fundamental as our entire civilization—surely does not show that the Government was meant to have the power to do so. Rather, as the Ninth Amendment expressly recognizes, there are fundamental personal rights such as this one, which are protected from abridgment by the Government though not specifically mentioned in the Constitution ...

The logic of the dissents would sanction federal or state legislation that seems to me even more plainly unconstitutional than the statute before us. Surely the Government, absent a showing of a compelling subordinating state interest, could not decree that all husbands and wives must be sterilized after two children have been born to them. Yet by their reasoning such an invasion of marital privacy would not be subject to constitutional challenge because, while it might be "silly," no provision of the Constitution specifically prevents the Government from curtailing the marital right to bear children and raise a family. While it may shock some of my Brethren that the Court today holds that the Constitution protects the right of marital privacy, in my view it is far more shocking to believe that the personal liberty guaranteed by the Constitution does not include protection against such totalitarian limitation of family size, which is at complete variance with our constitutional concepts. Yet, if upon a showing of a slender basis of rationality, a law outlawing voluntary birth control by married persons is valid, then, by the same reasoning, a law requiring compulsory birth control also would seem to be valid. In my view, however, both types of law would unjustifiably intrude upon rights of marital privacy which are constitutionally protected . . .

Although the Connecticut birth-control law obviously encroaches upon a fundamental personal liberty, the State does not show that the law serves any "subordinating [state] interest which is compelling" or that it is "necessary . . . to the accomplishment of a permissible state policy." The State, at most, argues that there is some rational relation between this statute and what is admittedly a legitimate subject of state concern—the discouraging of extra-marital relations. It says that preventing the use of birth-control devices by married persons helps prevent the indulgence by some in such extra-marital relations. The rationality of this justification is dubious, particularly in light of the admitted widespread availability to all persons in the State of Connecticut, unmarried as well as married, of birth-control devices for the prevention of disease, as distinguished from the prevention of conception. . . . But, in any event, it is clear that the state interest in safeguarding marital fidelity can be served by a more discriminately tailored statute, which does not, like the present one, sweep unnecessarily broadly, reaching far beyond the evil sought to be dealt with and intruding upon the privacy of all married couples. . . . Here, as elsewhere, "precision of regulation must be the touchstone in an area so closely touching our most precious freedoms." . . . The State of Connecticut does have statutes, the constitutionality of which is beyond doubt, which prohibit adultery and fornication. . . . These statutes demonstrate that means for achieving the same basic purpose of protecting marital fidelity are available to Connecticut without the need to "invade the area of protected freedoms." *NAACP v. Alabama* . . .

Finally, it should be said of the Court's holding today that it in no way interferes with a State's proper regulation of sexual promiscuity or misconduct. . . . "Adultery, homosexuality and the like are sexual intimacies which the State forbids . . . but the intimacy of husband and wife is necessarily an essential and accepted feature of the institution of marriage, an institution which the State not only must allow, but which always and in every age it has fostered and protected. It is one thing when the State exerts its power either to forbid extra-marital sexuality . . . or to say who may marry, but it is quite another when, having acknowledged a marriage and the intimacies inherent in it, it undertakes to regulate by means of the criminal law the details of that intimacy."

In sum, I believe that the right of privacy in the marital relation is fundamental and basic—a personal right "retained by the people" within the meaning of the Ninth Amendment. Connecticut cannot constitutionally abridge this fundamental right, which is protected by the Fourteenth Amendment from infringement by the States. I agree with the Court that petitioners' convictions must therefore be reversed.

MR. JUSTICE HARLAN, concurring in the judgment

I fully agree with the judgment of reversal, but find myself unable to join the Court's opinion. The reason is that it seems to me to evince an approach to this case very much like that taken by my Brothers BLACK and STEWART in dissent, namely: the Due Process Clause of the Fourteenth Amendment does not touch this Connecticut statute unless the enactment is found to violate some right assured by the letter or penumbra of the Bill of Rights.

In other words, what I find implicit in the Court's opinion is that the "incorporation" doctrine may be used to restrict the reach of Fourteenth Amendment Due Process. For me this is just as unacceptable constitutional doctrine as is the use of the "incorporation" approach to impose upon the States all the requirements of the Bill of Rights as found in the provisions of the first eight amendments and in the decisions of this Court interpreting them . . .

In my view, the proper constitutional inquiry in this case is whether this Connecticut statute infringes the Due Process Clause of the Fourteenth Amendment because the enactment violates basic values "implicit in the concept of ordered liberty," . . . I believe that it does . . .

While I could not more heartily agree that judicial "self restraint" is an indispensable ingredient of sound constitutional adjudication, I do submit that the formula suggested for achieving it is more hollow than real. "Specific" provisions of the Constitution, no less than "due process," lend themselves as readily to "personal" interpretations by judges whose constitutional outlook is simply to keep the Constitution in supposed "tune with the times" . . .

Judicial self-restraint will not, I suggest, be brought about in the "due process" area by the historically unfounded incorporation formula long advanced by my Brother BLACK, and now in part espoused by my Brother STEWART. It will be achieved in this area, as in other constitutional areas, only by continual insistence upon respect for the teachings of history, solid recognition of the basic values that underlie our society, and wise appreciation of the great roles that the doctrines of federalism and separation of powers have played in establishing and preserving American freedoms. . . . Adherence to these principles will not, of course, obviate all constitutional differences of opinion among judges, nor should it. Their continued recognition will, however, go farther toward keeping most judges from roaming at large in the constitutional field than will the interpolation into the Constitution of an artificial and largely illusory restriction on the content of the Due Process Clause.

MR. JUSTICE WHITE, concurring in the judgment

In my view this Connecticut law as applied to married couples deprives them of "liberty" without due process of law, as that concept is used in the Fourteenth Amendment. I therefore concur in the judgment of the Court reversing these convictions under Connecticut's aiding and abetting statute . . .

MR. JUSTICE BLACK, with whom MR. JUSTICE STEWART joins, dissenting

I agree with my Brother STEWART'S dissenting opinion. And like him I do not to any extent whatever base my view that this Connecticut law is constitutional on a belief that the law is wise or that its policy is a good one. In order that there may be no room at all to doubt why I vote as I do, I feel constrained to add that the law is every bit as offensive to me as it is to my Brethren of the majority and my Brothers HARLAN, WHITE and GOLDBERG who, reciting reasons why it is offensive to them, hold it unconstitutional. There is no single one of the graphic and eloquent strictures and criticisms fired at the policy of this Connecticut law either by the Court's opinion or by those of my concurring Brethren to which I cannot subscribe—except their conclusion that the evil qualities they see in the law make it unconstitutional.

Had the doctor defendant here, or even the nondoctor defendant, been convicted for doing nothing more than expressing opinions to persons coming to the clinic that certain contraceptive devices, medicines or practices would do them good and would be desirable, or for telling people how devices could be used, I can think of no reasons at this time why their expressions of views would not be protected by the First and Fourteenth Amendments, which guarantee freedom of speech. . . . But speech is one thing; conduct and physical activities are quite another. . . . The two defendants here were active participants in an organization which gave physical examinations to women, advised them what kind of contraceptive devices or medicines would most likely be satisfactory for them, and then supplied the devices themselves, all for a graduated scale of fees, based on the family income. Thus these defendants admittedly engaged with others in a planned course of conduct to help people violate the Connecticut law. Merely because some speech was used in carrying on that conduct—just as in ordinary life some speech accompanies most kinds of conduct—we are not in my view justified in holding that the First Amendment forbids the State to punish their conduct. Strongly as I desire to protect all First Amendment freedoms, I am unable to stretch the Amendment so as to afford protection to the conduct of these defendants in violating the Connecticut law. What would be the constitutional fate of the law if hereafter applied to punish nothing but speech is, as I have said, quite another matter.

The Court talks about a constitutional "right of privacy" as though there is some constitutional provision or provisions forbidding any law ever to be passed which might abridge the "privacy" of individuals. But there is not. There are, of course, guarantees in certain specific constitutional provisions which are designed in part to protect privacy at certain times and places with respect to certain activities. Such, for example, is the Fourth Amendment's guarantee against "unreasonable searches and seizures." But I think it belittles that Amendment to talk about it as though it protects nothing but "privacy." To treat it that way is to give it a niggardly interpretation, not the kind of liberal reading I think any Bill of Rights provision should be given. The average man would very likely not have his feelings soothed any more by having his property seized openly than by having it seized privately and by stealth. He simply wants his property left alone. And a person can be just as much, if not more, irritated, annoyed and injured by an unceremonious public arrest by a policeman as he is by a seizure in the privacy of his office or home.

One of the most effective ways of diluting or expanding a constitutionally guaranteed right is to substitute for the crucial word or words of a constitutional guarantee another word or words, more or less flexible and more or less restricted in meaning. This fact is well illustrated by the use of the term "right of privacy" as a comprehensive substitute for the Fourth Amendment's guarantee against "unreasonable searches and seizures." "Privacy" is a broad, abstract and ambiguous concept which can easily be shrunken in meaning but which can also, on the other hand, easily be interpreted as a constitutional ban against many things other than searches and seizures. I have expressed the view many times that First Amendment freedoms, for example, have suffered from a failure of the courts to stick to the simple language of the First Amendment in construing it, instead of invoking multitudes of words substituted for those the Framers used. . . . For these reasons I get nowhere in this case by talk about a constitutional "right of privacy" as an emanation from one or more constitutional provisions. I like my privacy as well as the next one, but I am nevertheless compelled to admit that government has a right to invade it unless prohibited by some specific constitutional provision. For these reasons I cannot agree with the Court's judgment and the reasons it gives for holding this Connecticut law unconstitutional . . .

The due process argument which my Brothers HARLAN and WHITE adopt here is based, as their opinions indicate, on the premise that this Court is vested with power to invalidate all state laws that it considers to be arbitrary, capricious, unreasonable, or oppressive, or on this Court's belief that a particular state law under scrutiny has no "rational or justifying" purpose, or is offensive to a "sense of fairness and justice." If these formulas based on "natural justice," or others which mean the same thing, are to prevail, they require judges to determine what is or is not constitutional on the basis of their own appraisal of what laws are unwise or unnecessary. The power to make such decisions is of course that of a legislative body. Surely it has to be admitted that no provision of the Constitution specifically gives such blanket power to courts to exercise such a supervisory veto over the wisdom and value of legislative policies and to hold unconstitutional those laws which they believe unwise or dangerous. I readily admit that no legislative body, state or national, should pass laws that can justly be given any of the invidious labels invoked as constitutional excuses to strike down state laws. But perhaps it is not too much to say that no legislative body ever does pass laws without believing that they will accomplish a sane, rational, wise and justifiable purpose. While I completely subscribe to the holding of *Marbury v. Madison* . . . and subsequent cases, that our Court has constitutional power to strike down statutes, state or federal, that violate commands of the Federal Constitution, I do not believe that we are granted power by the Due Process Clause or any other constitutional provision or provisions to measure constitutionality by our belief that legislation is arbitrary, capricious or unreasonable, or accomplishes no justifiable purpose, or is offensive to our own notions of "civilized standards of conduct." Such an appraisal of the wisdom of legislation is an attribute of the power to make laws, not of the power to interpret them. The use by federal courts of such a formula or doctrine or whatnot to veto federal or state laws simply takes away from Congress and States the power to make laws based on their own judgment of fairness and wisdom and transfers that power to this Court for ultimate determination—a power which was specifically denied to federal courts by the convention that framed the Constitution . . .

My Brother GOLDBERG has adopted the recent discovery that the Ninth Amendment as well as the Due Process Clause can be used by this Court as authority to strike down all state legislation which this Court thinks violates "fundamental principles of liberty and justice," or is contrary to the "traditions and [collective] conscience of our people." He also states, without proof satisfactory to me, that in making decisions on this basis judges will not consider "their personal and private notions." One may ask how they can avoid considering them. Our Court certainly has no machinery with which to take a Gallup Poll. And the scientific miracles of this age have not yet produced a gadget which the Court can use to determine what traditions are rooted in the "[collective] conscience of our people." Moreover, one would certainly have to look far beyond the language of the Ninth Amendment to find that the Framers vested in this Court any such awesome veto powers over lawmaking, either by the States or by the Congress. Nor does anything in the history of the Amendment offer any support for such a shocking doctrine. The whole history of the adoption of the Constitution and Bill of Rights points the other way, and the very material quoted by my Brother GOLDBERG shows that the Ninth Amendment was intended to protect against the idea that "by enumerating particular exceptions to the grant of power" to the Federal Government, "those rights which were not singled out, were intended to be assigned into the hands of the General Government [the United States], and were consequently insecure." That Amendment was passed, not to broaden the powers of this Court or any other department of "the General Government," but, as every student of history knows, to assure the people that the Constitution in all its provisions was intended to limit the Federal Government to the powers granted expressly or by necessary implication. If any broad, unlimited power to hold laws unconstitutional because they offend what this Court conceives to be the "[collective] conscience of our people" is vested in this Court by the Ninth Amendment, the Fourteenth Amendment, or any other provision of the Constitution, it was not given by the Framers, but rather has been bestowed on the Court by the Court. This fact is perhaps responsible for the peculiar phenomenon that for a period of a century and a half no serious suggestion was ever made that the Ninth Amendment, enacted to protect state powers against federal invasion, could be used as a weapon of federal power to prevent state legislatures from passing laws they consider appropriate to govern local affairs. Use of any such broad, unbounded judicial authority would make of this Court's members a day-to-day constitutional convention.

I repeat so as not to be misunderstood that this Court does have power, which it should exercise, to hold laws unconstitutional where they are forbidden by the Federal Constitution. My point is that there is no provision of the Constitution which either expressly or impliedly vests power in this Court to sit as a supervisory agency over acts of duly constituted legislative bodies and set aside their laws because of the Court's belief that the legislative policies adopted are unreasonable, unwise, arbitrary, capricious or irrational. The adoption of such a loose, flexible, uncontrolled standard for holding laws unconstitutional, if ever it is finally achieved, will amount to a great unconstitutional shift of power to the courts which I believe and am constrained to say will be bad for the courts and worse for the country. Subjecting federal and state laws to such an unrestrained and unrestrainable judicial control as to the wisdom of legislative enactments would, I fear, jeopardize the separation of governmental powers that the Framers set up and at the same time threaten to take away much of the power of States to govern themselves which the Constitution plainly intended them to have.

I realize that many good and able men have eloquently spoken and written, sometimes in rhapsodical strains, about the duty of this Court to keep the Constitution in tune with the times. The idea is that the Constitution must be changed from time to time and that this Court is charged with a duty to make those changes. For myself, I must with all deference reject that philosophy. The Constitution makers knew the need for change and provided for it. Amendments suggested by the people's elected representatives can be submitted to the people or their selected agents for ratification. That method of change was good for our Fathers, and being somewhat old-fashioned I must add it is good enough for me. And so, I cannot rely on the Due Process Clause or the Ninth Amendment or any mysterious and uncertain natural law concept as a reason for striking down this state law. The Due Process Clause with an "arbitrary and capricious" or "shocking to the conscience" formula was liberally used by this Court to strike down economic legislation in the early decades of this century, threatening, many people thought, the tranquility and stability of the Nation.... That formula, based on subjective considerations of "natural justice," is no less dangerous when used to enforce this Court's views about personal rights than those about economic rights. I had thought that we had laid that formula, as a means for striking down state legislation, to rest once and for all . . .

In 1798, when this Court was asked to hold another Connecticut law unconstitutional, Justice Iredell said:

"It has been the policy of all the American states, which have, individually, framed their state constitutions since the revolution, and of the people of the United States, when they framed the Federal Constitution, to define with precision the objects of the legislative power, and to restrain its exercise within marked and settled boundaries. If any act of Congress, or of the Legislature of a state, violates those constitutional provisions, it is unquestionably void; though, I admit, that as the authority to declare it void is of a delicate and awful nature, the Court will never resort to that authority, but in a clear and urgent case. If, on the other hand, the Legislature of the Union, or the Legislature of any member of the Union, shall pass a law, within the general scope of their constitutional power, the Court cannot pronounce it to be void, merely because it is, in their judgment, contrary to the principles of natural justice. The ideas of natural justice are regulated by no fixed standard: the ablest and the purest men have differed upon the subject; and all that the Court could properly say, in such an event, would be, that the Legislature (possessed of an equal right of opinion) had passed an act which, in the opinion of the judges, was inconsistent with the abstract principles of natural justice." *Calder v. Bull.*

I would adhere to that constitutional philosophy in passing on this Connecticut law today. I am not persuaded to deviate from the view . . .

The late Judge Learned Hand, after emphasizing his view that judges should not use the due process formula suggested in the concurring opinions today or any other formula like it to invalidate legislation offensive to their "personal preferences," made the statement, with which I fully agree, that:

"For myself it would be most irksome to be ruled by a bevy of Platonic Guardians, even if I knew how to choose them, which I assuredly do not."

So far as I am concerned, Connecticut's law as applied here is not forbidden by any provision of the Federal Constitution as that Constitution was written, and I would therefore affirm.

MR. JUSTICE STEWART, whom MR. JUSTICE BLACK joins, dissenting

Since 1879 Connecticut has had on its books a law which forbids the use of contraceptives by anyone. I think this is an uncommonly silly law. As a practical matter, the law is obviously unenforceable, except in the oblique context of the present case. As a philosophical matter, I believe the use of contraceptives in the relationship of marriage should be left to personal and private choice, based upon each individual's moral, ethical, and religious beliefs. As a matter of social policy, I think professional counsel about methods of birth control should be available to all, so that each individual's choice can be meaningfully made. But we are not asked in this case to say whether we think this law is unwise, or even asinine. We are asked to hold that it violates the United States Constitution. And that I cannot do.

In the course of its opinion the Court refers to no less than six Amendments to the Constitution: the First, the Third, the Fourth, the Fifth, the Ninth, and the Fourteenth. But the Court does not say which of these Amendments, if any, it thinks is infringed by this Connecticut law.

We are told that the Due Process Clause of the Fourteenth Amendment is not, as such, the "guide" in this case. With that much I agree. There is no claim that this law, duly enacted by the Connecticut Legislature, is unconstitutionally vague. There is no claim that the appellants were denied any of the elements of procedural due process at their trial, so as to make their convictions constitutionally invalid. And, as the Court says, the day has long passed since the Due Process Clause was regarded as a proper instrument for determining "the wisdom, need, and propriety" of state laws . . .

As to the First, Third, Fourth, and Fifth Amendments, I can find nothing in any of them to invalidate this Connecticut law, even assuming that all those Amendments are fully applicable against the States. It has not even been argued that this is a law "respecting an establishment of religion, or prohibiting the free exercise thereof." And surely, unless the solemn process of constitutional adjudication is to descend to the level of a play on words, there is not involved here any abridgment of "the freedom of speech, or of the press; or the right of the people peaceably to assemble, and to petition the Government for a redress of grievances." No soldier has been quartered in any house. There has been no search, and no seizure. Nobody has been compelled to be a witness against himself.

The Court also quotes the Ninth Amendment, and my Brother GOLDBERG's concurring opinion relies heavily upon it. But to say that the Ninth Amendment has anything to do with this case is to turn somersaults with history. The Ninth Amendment, like its companion the Tenth, which this Court held "states but a truism that all is retained which has not been surrendered," *United States v. Darby* . . . was framed by James Madison and adopted by the States simply to make clear that the adoption of the Bill of Rights did not alter the plan that the Federal Government was to be a government of express and limited powers, and that all rights and powers not delegated to it were retained by the people and the individual States. Until today no member of this Court has ever suggested that the Ninth Amendment meant anything else, and the idea that a federal court could ever use the Ninth Amendment to annul a law passed by the elected representatives of the people of the State of Connecticut would have caused James Madison no little wonder.

What provision of the Constitution, then, does make this state law invalid? The Court says it is the right of privacy "created by several fundamental constitutional guarantees." With all deference, I can find no such general right of privacy in the Bill of Rights, in any other part of the Constitution, or in any case ever before decided by this Court.

At the oral argument in this case we were told that the Connecticut law does not "conform to current community standards." But it is not the function of this Court to decide cases on the basis of community standards. We are here to decide cases "agreeably to the Constitution and laws of the United States." It is the essence of judicial duty to subordinate our own personal views, our own ideas of what legislation is wise and what is not. If, as I should surely hope, the law before us does not reflect the standards of the people of Connecticut, the people of Connecticut can freely exercise their true Ninth and Tenth Amendment rights to persuade their elected representatives to repeal it. That is the constitutional way to take this law off the books.

Religious Reactions—Free Choice or Intrinsic Evil?

In 1968, the Catholic Church stood alone as the only dominant religious body in the United States to continue its prohibitions of birth control. The publication of Humanae Vitae *created considerable divisions between the Church and society, prompting some policymakers to dismiss the Catholic voice as too far out of line with popular consensus. The encyclical also prompted vocal divisions within the Church itself between the laity, priests, and some bishops. The key question at issue was whether certain practices arising from modern science necessarily involve the offices of the Church. Does the morality of birth control depend on the circumstances of each individual? If so, then it is a matter of free choice and not a matter for Church oversight. Or is the practice of artificial birth control an intrinsically evil act? If so, then the practice is prohibited by the Church for the same reasons that abortion and euthanasia are condemned.*

The following selection is an excerpt from the 1968 encyclical Humanae Vitae, *which states explicitly that birth control is an intrinsic evil.*

EXCERPT FROM *HUMANAE VITAE*

Pope Paul VI, *Humanae Vitae: On The Regulation of Birth* (1968) (c) Libreria Editrice Vaticana, used by permission.

During the Second Vatican Council, Pope John XXIII called a special papal commission to consider the moral implications of artificial contraception. After more than five years of discussion, the commission recommended that the Church consider avenues for tolerating artificial methods of regulating birth. Pope Paul VI, however, chose not to follow the recommendation and instead reaffirmed the Church's traditional teaching on the subject. He argues that birth control, sterilization, and abortion are all intrinsically evil acts.

By 1968, the Catholic Church was less concerned by eugenics based arguments than it had been in 1930. Instead, the pope devotes more time refuting pro-contraception argument based on population control and women's rights. Since birth control was no longer viewed as a matter of obscenity, what basis did the Catholic Church continue to oppose artificial contraception? How does that basis differ from earlier presumptions of the temperance movement?

The transmission of human life is a most serious role in which married people collaborate freely and responsibly with God the Creator. It has always been a source of great joy to them, even though it sometimes entails many difficulties and hardships.

The fulfillment of this duty has always posed problems to the conscience of married people, but the recent course of human society and the concomitant changes have provoked new questions. The Church cannot ignore these questions, for they concern matters intimately connected with the life and happiness of human beings . . .

2. The changes that have taken place are of considerable importance and varied in nature. In the first place there is the rapid increase in population which has made many fear that world population is going to grow faster than available resources, with the consequence that many families and developing countries would be faced with greater hardships. This can easily induce public authorities to be tempted to take even harsher measures to avert this danger. There is also the fact that not only working and housing conditions but the greater demands made both in the economic and educational field pose a living situation in which it is frequently difficult these days to provide properly for a large family.

Also noteworthy is a new understanding of the dignity of woman and her place in society, of the value of conjugal love in marriage and the relationship of conjugal acts to this love.

But the most remarkable development of all is to be seen in man's stupendous progress in the domination and rational organization of the forces of nature to the point that he is endeavoring to extend this control over every aspect of his own life—over his body, over his mind and emotions, over his social life, and even over the laws that regulate the transmission of life . . .

Special Studies

5. The consciousness of the same responsibility induced Us to confirm and expand the commission set up by Our predecessor Pope John XXIII, of happy memory, in March, 1963. This commission included married couples as well as many experts in the various fields pertinent to these questions. Its task was to examine views and opinions concerning married life, and especially on the correct regulation of births; and it was also to provide the teaching authority of the Church with such evidence as would enable it to give an apt reply in this matter, which not only the faithful but also the rest of the world were waiting for . . .

The Magisterium's Reply

6. However, the conclusions arrived at by the commission could not be considered by Us as definitive and absolutely certain, dispensing Us from the duty of examining personally this serious question. This was all the more necessary because, within the commission itself, there was not complete agreement concerning the moral norms to be proposed, and especially because certain approaches and criteria for a solution to this question had emerged which were at variance with the moral doctrine on marriage constantly taught by the magisterium of the Church . . .

II. DOCTRINAL PRINCIPLES

7. The question of human procreation, like every other question which touches human life, involves more than the limited aspects specific to such disciplines as biology, psychology, demography or sociology. It is the whole man and the whole mission to which he is called that must be considered: both its natural, earthly aspects and its supernatural, eternal aspects. And since in the attempt to justify artificial methods of birth control many appeal to the demands of married love or of responsible parenthood, these two important realities of married life must be accurately defined and analyzed . . .

God's Loving Design

8. Marriage, then, is far from being the effect of chance or the result of the blind evolution of natural forces. It is in reality the wise and provident institution of God the Creator, whose purpose was to effect in man His loving design. As a consequence, husband and wife, through that mutual gift of themselves, which is specific and exclusive to them alone, develop that union of two persons in which they perfect one another, cooperating with God in the generation and rearing of new lives . . .

Married Love

9. In the light of these facts the characteristic features and exigencies of married love are clearly indicated, and it is of the highest importance to evaluate them exactly.

This love is above all fully human, a compound of sense and spirit. It is not, then, merely a question of natural instinct or emotional drive. It is also, and above all, an act of the free will, whose trust is such that it is meant not only to survive the joys and sorrows of daily life, but also to grow, so that husband and wife become in a way one heart and one soul, and together attain their human fulfillment . . .

Married love is also faithful and exclusive of all other, and this until death. This is how husband and wife understood it on the day on which, fully aware of what they were doing, they freely vowed themselves to one another in marriage . . .

Finally, this love is fecund. It is not confined wholly to the loving interchange of husband and wife; it also contrives to go beyond this to bring new life into being. "Marriage and conjugal love are by their nature ordained toward the procreation and education of children. Children are really the supreme gift of marriage and contribute in the highest degree to their parents' welfare."

Responsible Parenthood

10. Married love, therefore, requires of husband and wife the full awareness of their obligations in the matter of responsible parenthood, which today, rightly enough, is much insisted upon, but which at the same time should be rightly understood. Thus, we do well to consider responsible parenthood in the light of its varied legitimate and interrelated aspects . . .

Responsible parenthood, as we use the term here, has one further essential aspect of paramount importance. It concerns the objective moral order which was established by God, and of which a right conscience is the true interpreter. In a word, the exercise of responsible parenthood requires that husband and wife, keeping a right order of priorities, recognize their own duties toward God, themselves, their families and human society.

From this it follows that they are not free to act as they choose in the service of transmitting life, as if it were wholly up to them to decide what is the right course to follow. On the contrary, they are bound to ensure that what they do corresponds to the will of God the Creator. The very nature of marriage and its use makes His will clear, while the constant teaching of the Church spells it out . . .

Observing the Natural Law

11. The fact is, as experience shows, that new life is not the result of each and every act of sexual intercourse. God has wisely ordered laws of nature and the incidence of fertility in such a way that successive births are already naturally spaced through the inherent operation of these laws. The Church, nevertheless, in urging men to the observance of the precepts of the natural law, which it interprets by its constant doctrine, teaches that each and every marital act must of necessity retain its intrinsic relationship to the procreation of human life.

Union and Procreation

12. This particular doctrine, often expounded by the magisterium of the Church, is based on the inseparable connection, established by God, which man on his own initiative may not break, between the unitive significance and the procreative significance which are both inherent to the marriage act.

The reason is that the fundamental nature of the marriage act, while uniting husband and wife in the closest intimacy, also renders them capable of generating new life—and this as a result of laws written into the actual nature of man and of woman. And if each of these essential qualities, the unitive and the procreative, is preserved, the use of marriage fully retains its sense of true mutual love and its ordination to the supreme responsibility of parenthood to which man is called. We believe that our contemporaries are particularly capable of seeing that this teaching is in harmony with human reason.

Faithfulness to God's Design

13. Men rightly observe that a conjugal act imposed on one's partner without regard to his or her condition or personal and reasonable wishes in the matter, is no true act of love, and therefore offends the moral order in its particular application to the intimate relationship of husband and wife. If they further reflect, they must also recognize that an act of mutual love which impairs the capacity to transmit life which God the Creator, through specific laws, has built into it, frustrates His design which constitutes the norm of marriage, and contradicts the will of the Author of life. Hence to use this divine gift while depriving it, even if only partially, of its meaning and purpose, is equally repugnant to the nature of man and of woman, and is consequently in opposition to the plan of God and His holy will. But to experience the gift of married love while respecting the laws of conception is to acknowledge that one is not the master of the sources of life but rather the minister of the design established by the Creator. Just as man does not have unlimited dominion over his body in general, so also, and with more particular reason, he has no such dominion over his specifically sexual faculties, for these are concerned by their very nature with the generation of life, of which God is the source. "Human life is sacred—all men must recognize that fact," Our predecessor Pope John XXIII recalled. "From its very inception it reveals the creating hand of God."

Unlawful Birth Control Methods

14. Therefore We base Our words on the first principles of a human and Christian doctrine of marriage when We are obliged once more to declare that the direct interruption of the generative process already begun and, above all, all direct abortion, even for therapeutic reasons, are to be absolutely excluded as lawful means of regulating the number of children. Equally to be condemned, as the magisterium of the Church has affirmed on many occasions, is direct sterilization, whether of the man or of the woman, whether permanent or temporary. Similarly excluded is any action which either before, at the moment of, or after sexual intercourse, is specifically intended to prevent procreation—whether as an end or as a means . . .

Lawful Therapeutic Means

15. On the other hand, the Church does not consider at all illicit the use of those therapeutic means necessary to cure bodily diseases, even if a foreseeable impediment to procreation should result there from—provided such impediment is not directly intended for any motive whatsoever.

Recourse to Infertile Periods

16. Now as We noted earlier (no. 3), some people today raise the objection against this particular doctrine of the Church concerning the moral laws governing marriage, that human intelligence has both the right and responsibility to control those forces of irrational nature which come within its ambit and to direct them toward ends beneficial to man. Others ask on the same point whether it is not reasonable in so many cases to use artificial birth control if by so doing the harmony and peace of a family are better served and more suitable conditions are provided for the education of children already born. To this question We must give a clear reply. The Church is the first to praise and commend the application of human intelligence to an activity in which a rational creature such as man is so closely associated with his Creator. But she affirms that this must be done within the limits of the order of reality established by God.

If therefore there are well-grounded reasons for spacing births, arising from the physical or psychological condition of husband or wife, or from external circumstances, the Church teaches that married people may then take advantage of the natural cycles immanent in the reproductive system and engage in marital intercourse only during those times that are infertile, thus controlling birth in a way which does not in the least offend the moral principles which We have just explained.

Neither the Church nor her doctrine is inconsistent when she considers it lawful for married people to take advantage of the infertile period but condemns as always unlawful the use of means which directly prevent conception, even when the reasons given for the later practice may appear to be upright and serious. In reality, these two cases are completely different. In the former the married couple rightly use a faculty provided them by nature. In the latter they obstruct the natural development of the generative process. It cannot be denied that in each case the married couple, for acceptable reasons, are both perfectly clear in their intention to avoid children and wish to make sure that none will result. But it is equally true that it is exclusively in the former case that husband and wife are ready to abstain from intercourse during the fertile period as often as for reasonable motives the birth of another child is not desirable. And when the infertile period recurs, they use their married intimacy to express their mutual love and safeguard their fidelity toward one another. In doing this they certainly give proof of a true and authentic love.

Consequences of Artificial Methods

17. Responsible men can become more deeply convinced of the truth of the doctrine laid down by the Church on this issue if they reflect on the consequences of methods and plans for artificial birth control. Let them first consider how easily this course of action could open wide the way for marital infidelity and a general lowering of moral standards. Not much experience is needed to be fully aware of human weakness and to understand that human beings—and especially the

young, who are so exposed to temptation—need incentives to keep the moral law, and it is an evil thing to make it easy for them to break that law. Another effect that gives cause for alarm is that a man who grows accustomed to the use of contraceptive methods may forget the reverence due to a woman, and, disregarding her physical and emotional equilibrium, reduce her to being a mere instrument for the satisfaction of his own desires, no longer considering her as his partner whom he should surround with care and affection.

Finally, careful consideration should be given to the danger of this power passing into the hands of those public authorities who care little for the precepts of the moral law. Who will blame a government which in its attempt to resolve the problems affecting an entire country resorts to the same measures as are regarded as lawful by married people in the solution of a particular family difficulty? Who will prevent public authorities from favoring those contraceptive methods which they consider more effective? Should they regard this as necessary, they may even impose their use on everyone. It could well happen, therefore, that when people, either individually or in family or social life, experience the inherent difficulties of the divine law and are determined to avoid them, they may give into the hands of public authorities the power to intervene in the most personal and intimate responsibility of husband and wife.

Limits to Man's Power

Consequently, unless we are willing that the responsibility of procreating life should be left to the arbitrary decision of men, we must accept that there are certain limits, beyond which it is wrong to go, to the power of man over his own body and its natural functions—limits, let it be said, which no one, whether as a private individual or as a public authority, can lawfully exceed . . .

Concern of the Church

18. It is to be anticipated that perhaps not everyone will easily accept this particular teaching. There is too much clamorous outcry against the voice of the Church, and this is intensified by modern means of communication. But it comes as no surprise to the Church that she, no less than her divine Founder, is destined to be a "sign of contradiction." She does not, because of this, evade the duty imposed on her of proclaiming humbly but firmly the entire moral law, both natural and evangelical.

Since the Church did not make either of these laws, she cannot be their arbiter—only their guardian and interpreter. It could never be right for her to declare lawful what is in fact unlawful, since that, by its very nature, is always opposed to the true good of man. In preserving intact the whole moral law of marriage, the Church is convinced that she is contributing to the creation of a truly human civilization. She urges man not to betray his personal responsibilities by putting all his faith in technical expedients. In this way she defends the dignity of husband and wife.

This course of action shows that the Church, loyal to the example and teaching of the divine Savior, is sincere and unselfish in her regard for men whom she strives to help even now during this earthly pilgrimage "to share God's life as sons of the living God, the Father of all men." . . .

III. PASTORAL DIRECTIVES

Value of Self-Discipline

21. The right and lawful ordering of birth demands, first of all, that spouses fully recognize and value the true blessings of family life and that they acquire complete mastery over themselves and their emotions. For if with the aid of reason and of free will they are to control their natural drives, there can be no doubt at all of the need for self-denial. Only then will the expression of love, essential to married life, conform to right order. This is especially clear in the practice of periodic continence. Self-discipline of this kind is a shining witness to the chastity of husband and wife and, far from being a hindrance to their love of one another, transforms it by giving it a more truly human character. And if this self-discipline does demand that they persevere in their purpose and efforts, it has at the same time the salutary effect of enabling husband and wife to develop to their personalities and to be enriched with spiritual blessings. For it brings to family life abundant fruits of tranquility and peace. It helps in solving difficulties of other kinds. It fosters in husband and wife thoughtfulness and loving consideration for one another. It helps them to repel inordinate self-love, which is the opposite of charity. It arouses in them a consciousness of their responsibilities. And finally, it confers upon parents a deeper and more effective influence in the education of their children. As their children grow up, they develop a right sense of values and achieve a serene and harmonious use of their mental and physical powers.

Promotion of Chastity

22. We take this opportunity to address those who are engaged in education and all those whose right and duty it is to provide for the common good of human society. We would call their attention to the need to create an atmosphere favorable to the growth of chastity so that true liberty may prevail over license and the norms of the moral law may be fully safeguarded. Everything therefore in the modern means of social communication which arouses men's baser passions and encourages low moral standards, as well as every obscenity in the written word and every form of indecency on the stage and screen, should be condemned publicly and unanimously by all those who have at heart the advance of civilization and the safeguarding of the outstanding values of the human spirit. It is quite absurd to defend this kind of depravity in the name of art or culture or by pleading the liberty which may be allowed in this field by the public authorities.

Birth Control as a Political Issue—Is Abortion a Form of Birth Control?

In 1984, President Ronald Reagan announced a change in American foreign aid policy while at the UN International Conference on Population held in Mexico City. Previously, American foreign aid that was intended to promote family planning did not distinguish between recipient clinics that provided contraceptives and those that provided abortions. In the United States, the Hyde Amendment prohibited use of federal funds to pay for abortion services. The disposition of foreign aid for humanitarian purposes was left largely to the jurisdiction of the executive branch and not the legislature. As such, the Hyde Amendment had no impact on federal monies spent outside the United States. President Reagan announced that he would use an executive order to specifically prohibit use of American aid for abortion services overseas. In effect, he was applying the Hyde Amendment to foreign aid.

Since 1984, the question of whether American foreign aid should be used for abortion services has been known as the "Mexico City Policy." Each president of a successive party has used his election to reverse the Mexico City Policy of his predecessor. Democrats have rescinded the policy, while Republicans have reinstated it. President Bill Clinton reversed Reagan's policy, President George W. Bush reinstated it, and President Barack Obama reversed Bush's policy.

The fundamental question that divided the partisan positions on the Mexico City Policy is whether abortion should be included as a form of family planning, birth control, and other contraceptive services. Since the first introduction of a "Hyde Amendment" in 1977, Republican presidents have consistently argued that abortion was a separate kind of procedure and should not be treated as a form of birth control. For their part, Democratic presidents have consistently argued the opposite. Included in the following selections are executive orders of each president since Ronald Reagan relating to Mexico City Policy.

HYDE AMENDMENT

H.Amdt.185 (A008) to bill H.R. 2518, 103rd Congress, June 30th, 1993.

The First "Hyde Amendment" was introduced by Illinois Congressmen Henry J. Hyde in 1976. It was a short rider attached to Health and Human Services appropriations bills that prohibited the use of federal monies for abortion services. After the initial introduction, Republicans routinely attached the amendment to all appropriations bills that might involve practice, instruction, and recommendations for abortion services.

Despite the legality of abortion in every state, the Supreme Court affirmed the federal legislature's right to distinguish abortion from other medical procedures. In 1980, the Court ruled in Harris v. McRae *that abortion involved the "purposeful termination of a potential life" and was thus inherently different from other medical procedures. The Republican and Democratic party platforms continue to disagree on this point.*

In 1980, the Hyde Amendment read:

None of the funds appropriated under this Act shall be used to perform abortions except where the life of the mother would be endangered if the fetus were carried to term.

In 1993, abortion advocates threatened to build a political coalition that would eliminate the Hyde Amendment unless specific exceptions were inserted to account for cases of rape, incest, or risk to the life of the mother. The 1993 version of the Hyde Amendment read:

None of the funds appropriated under this Act shall be expended for any abortion except when it is made known to the federal entity or official to which funds are appropriated under this Act that such procedure is necessary to save the life of the mother or that the pregnancy is the result of an act of rape or incest.

REAGAN'S MEXICO CITY POLICY

Policy Statement of the United States of America at the United Nations International Conference on Population (Second Session) Mexico, D.F., August 6–14, 1984.
Policy Statement: International Conference on Population.

Introduction

For many years, the United States has supported, and helped to finance, programs of family planning, particularly in developing countries. This

Administration has continued that support but has placed it within a policy context different from that of the past. It is sufficiently evident that the current exponential growth in global population cannot continue indefinitely. There is no question of the ultimate need to achieve a condition of population equilibrium. The differences that do exist concern the choice of strategies and methods for the achievement of that goal. The experience of the last two decades not only makes possible but requires a sharper focus for our population policy. It requires a more refined approach to problems which appear today in quite a different light than they did twenty years ago.

First and most important, population growth is, of itself, a neutral phenomenon. It is not necessarily good or ill. It becomes an asset or a problem only in conjunction with other factors, such as economic policy, social constraints, need for manpower, and so forth. The relationship between population growth and economic development is not necessarily a negative one. More people do not necessarily mean less growth. Indeed, in the economic history of many nations, population growth has been an essential element in economic progress.

Before the advent of governmental population programs, several factors had combined to create an unprecedented surge in population over most of the world. Although population levels in many industrialized nations had reached or were approaching equilibrium in the period before the Second World War, the baby boom that followed in its wake resulted in a dramatic, but temporary, population "tilt" toward youth. The disproportionate number of infants, children, teenagers, and eventually young adults, did strain the social infrastructure of schools, health facilities, law enforcement, and so forth. However, it also helped sustain strong economic growth, despite occasionally counterproductive government policies.

Among the developing nations, a coincidental population increase was caused by entirely different factors. A tremendous expansion of health services—from simple inoculations to sophisticated surgery—saved millions of lives every year. Emergency relief, facilitated by modern transport, helped millions to survive flood, famine, and drought, The sharing of technology, the teaching of agriculture and engineering and improvements in educational standards generally, all helped to reduce mortality rates, especially infant mortality, and to lengthen life spans.

This demonstrated not poor planning or bad policy but human progress in a new era of international assistance, technological advance, and human compassion. The population boom was a challenge; it need not have been a crisis. Seen in its broader context, it required a measured, modulated response. It provoked an overreaction by some, largely, because it coincided with two negative factors which, together, hindered families and nations in adapting to their changing circumstances.

The first of these factors was governmental control of economies, a development which effectively constrained economic growth. The post-war experience consistently demonstrated that, as economic decision-making was concentrated in the hands of planners and public officials, the ability of average men and women to work towards a better future was impaired, and sometimes crippled. In many cases, agriculture was devastated by government price-fixing that wiped out rewards for labor. Job creation in infant industries was hampered by confiscatory taxes. Personal industry and thrift were penalized, while dependence upon the state was encouraged. Political considerations made it difficult for an economy to adjust to changes in supply and demand or to disruptions in world trade and finance. Under such circumstances, population growth changed from an asset in the development of economic potential to a peril.

One of the consequences of this "economic statism" was that it disrupted the natural mechanism for slowing population growth in problem areas. The world's more affluent nations have reached a population equilibrium without compulsion and, in most cases, even before it was government policy to achieve it. The controlling factor in these cases has been the adjustment, by individual families, of reproductive behavior to economic opportunity and aspiration. Historically, as opportunities and the standard of living rise, the birth rate falls. In many countries, economic freedom has led to economically rational behavior.

That pattern might be well under way in many nations where population growth is today a problem, if counterproductive government policies had not disrupted economic incentives, rewards, and advancement. In this regard, localized crises of population growth are, in part, evidence of too much government control and planning, rather than too little.

The second factor that turned the population boom into a crisis was confined to the western world. It was an outbreak of an anti-intellectualism, which attacked science, technology, and the very concept of material progress. Joined to a commendable and long overdue concern for the environment, it was more a reflection of anxiety about unsettled times and an uncertain future. In its disregard of human experience and scientific sophistication, it was not unlike other waves of cultural anxiety that have swept through western civilization during times of social stress and scientific exploration.

The combination of these two factors—counterproductive economic policies in poor and struggling nations, and a pessimism among the more advanced—led to a demographic overreaction in the 1960's and 1970's. Scientific forecasts were required to compete with unsound, extremist scenarios, and too many governments pursued population control measures without sound economic policies that create the rise in living standards historically associated with decline in fertility rates. This approach has not worked, primarily because it has focused on a symptom and neglected the underlying ailments. For the last three years, this Administration has sought to reverse that approach. We recognize that, in some cases, immediate population pressures may require short-term efforts to ameliorate them. But population control programs alone cannot substitute for the economic reforms that put a society on the road toward growth and, as an aftereffect, toward slower population increase as well.

Nor can population control substitute for the rapid and responsible development of natural resources. In commenting on the Global 2000 report, this

Administration in 1981 disagreed with its call for more governmental supervision and control, stating that:

"Historically, that has tended to restrict the availability of resources and to hamper the development of technology, rather than to assist it. Recognizing the seriousness of environmental and economic problems, and their relationship to social and political pressures, especially in the developing nations, the Administration places a priority upon technological advance and economic expansion, which hold out the hope of prosperity and stability of a rapidly changing world. That hope can be realized, of course, only to the extent that government's response to problems, whether economic or ecological, respects and enhances individual freedom, which make true progress possible and worthwhile."

Those principles underlie this country's approach to the International Conference on Population to be held in Mexico City in August.

Policy Objectives

The world's rapid population growth is a recent phenomenon. Only several decades ago, the population of developing countries was relatively stable, the result of a balance between high fertility and high mortality. There are now 4.5 billion people in the world, and six billion are projected by the year 2000. Such rapid growth places tremendous pressures on governments without concomitant economic growth.

The International Conference on Population offers the U.S. an opportunity to strengthen the international consensus on the interrelationships between economic development and population, which has emerged since the last such conference in Bucharest in 1974. Our primary objective will be to encourage developing countries to adopt sound economic policies and, where appropriate, population policies consistent with respect for human dignity and family values. As President Reagan stated in his message to the Mexico City Conference:

"We believe population programs can and must be truly voluntary, cognizant of the rights and responsibilities of individuals and families, and respectful of religious and cultural values. When they are, such programs can make an important contribution to economic and social development, to the health of mothers and children, and to the stability of the family and of society."

U.S. support for family planning programs is based on respect for human life, enhancement of human dignity, and strengthening of the family. Attempts to use abortion, involuntary sterilization, or other coercive measures in family planning must be shunned, whether exercised against families within a society or against nations within the family of man.

The United Nations Declaration of the Rights of the Child (1959) calls for legal protection for children before birth as well as after birth. In keeping with this obligation, the United States does not consider abortion an acceptable element of family planning programs and will no longer contribute to those of which it is a part. Accordingly, when dealing with nations which support abortion with funds not provided by the United States Government, the United States will contribute to such nations through segregated accounts which cannot be used for abortion. Moreover, the United States will no longer contribute to separate non-governmental organizations which perform or actively promote abortion as a method of family planning in other nations. With regard to the United Nations Fund for Population Activities (UNFPA), the U.S. will insist that no part of its contribution be used for abortion. The U.S. will also call for concrete assurances that the UNFPA is not engaged in, or does not provide funding for, abortion or coercive family planning programs; if such assurances are not forthcoming, the U.S. will redirect the amount of its contribution to other, non-UNFPA, family planning programs.

In addition, when efforts to lower population growth are deemed advisable, U.S. policy considers it imperative that such efforts respect the religious beliefs and culture of each society, and the right of couples to determine the size of heir own families. Accordingly, the U.S. will not provide family planning funds to any nation which engages in forcible coercion to achieve population growth objectives.

U.S. Government authorities will immediately begin negotiations to implement the above policies with the appropriate governments and organizations.

It is time to put additional emphasis upon those root problems which frequently exacerbate population pressures, but which have too often been given scant attention. By focusing upon real remedies for underdeveloped' economies, the International Conference on Population can reduce demographic issues to their proper place. It is an important place, but not the controlling one. It requires our continuing attention within the broader context of economic growth and of the economic freedom that is its prerequisite.

Population, Development, and Economic Policies

Conservative projections indicate that, in the sixty years from 1950 to 2010, many Third World countries will experience four-, five-, or even six-fold increases in the size of their populations. Even under the assumption of gradual declines in birth rates, the unusually high proportion of youth in the Third World means that the annual population growth in many of these countries will continue to increase for the next several decades.

Sound economic policies and a market economy are of fundamental importance to the process of economic development. Rising standards of living contributed in a major way to the demographic transition from high to low rates of population growth which occurred in the U.S. and other industrialized countries over the last century.

The current situation of many developing countries, however, differs in certain ways from conditions in 19th century Europe and the U.S. The rates and dimensions of population growth are much higher now, the pressures on land, water, and resources are greater, the safety-valve of migration is more restricted, and, perhaps most important, time is not on their side because of the momentum of demographic change.

Rapid population growth compounds already serious problems faced by both public and private sectors in accommodating changing social and economic demands. It diverts resources from needed investment, and increases the costs and difficulties of economic development. Slowing population growth is not a panacea for the problems of social and economic development. It is not offered as a substitute for sound and comprehensive development policies which encourage a vital private sector, it cannot solve problems of hunger, unemployment, crowding, or social disorder.

Population assistance is an ingredient of a comprehensive program that focuses on the root causes of development failures. The U.S. program as a whole, including population assistance, lays the basis for well-grounded, step-by-step initiatives to improve the well-being of people in developing countries and to make their own efforts, particularly through expanded private sector initiatives, a key building block of development programs.

Fortunately, a broad international consensus has emerged since the 1974 Bucharest World Population Conference that economic development and population policies are mutually reinforcing.

By helping developing countries slow their population growth through support for effective voluntary family planning programs, in conjunction with sound economic policies, U.S. population assistance contributes to stronger saving and investment rates, speeds the development of effective markets and related employment opportunities, reduces the potential resource requirements of programs to improve the health and education of the people, and hastens the achievement of each country's graduation from the need for external assistance.

The United States will continue its long-standing commitment to development assistance, of which population programs are a part. We recognize the importance of providing our assistance within the cultural, economic, and political context of the countries we are assisting, and in keeping with our own values.

Health and Humanitarian Concerns

Perhaps the most poignant consequence of rapid population growth is its effect on the health of mothers and children. Especially in poor countries, the health and nutrition status of women and children is linked to family size. Maternal and infant mortality rises with the number of births and with births too closely spaced. In countries as different as Turkey, Peru, and Nepal, a child born less than two years after its sibling is twice as likely to die before it reaches the age of five, than if there were an interval of at least four years between the births. Complications of pregnancy are more frequent among women who are very young or near the end of their reproductive years. In societies with widespread malnutrition and inadequate health conditions, these problems are reinforced; numerous and closely spaced births lead to even greater malnutrition of mothers and infants.

It is an unfortunate reality that, in many countries, abortion is used as a means of terminating unwanted pregnancies. This is unnecessary and repugnant; voluntary family assistance programs can provide a humane alternative to abortion for couples who wish to regulate the size of their family, and evidence from some developing countries indicates a decline in abortion as such services become available.

The basic objective of all U.S. assistance, including population programs, is the betterment of the human condition—improving the quality of life of mothers and children, of families, and of communities for generations to come. For we recognize that people are the ultimate resource—but this means happy and healthy children, growing up with education, finding productive work as young adults, and able to develop their full mental and physical potential.

U.S. aid is designed to promote economic progress in developing countries through encouraging sound economic policies and freeing of individual initiative. Thus, the U.S. supports a broad range of activities in various sectors, including agriculture, private enterprise, science and technology, health, population, and education. Population assistance amounts to about ten percent of total development assistance.

Technology as a Key to Development

The transfer, adaptation, and improvement of modern know-how is central to U.S. development assistance. People with greater know-how are people better able to improve their lives. Population assistance ensures that a wide range of modern demographic technology is made available to developing countries and that technological improvements critical for successful development receive support.

The efficient collection, processing, and analysis of data derived from census, survey, and vital statistics programs contribute to better planning in both the public and private sectors.

PRESIDENT WILLIAM CLINTON'S MEXICO CITY POLICY

Memorandum on the Mexico City Policy.
January 22, 1993. *Weekly Compilation of Presidential Documents* 29, no. 3: 88. Washington, DC: Office of the Federal Register (OFR), National Archives and Records Administration (NARA).

Memorandum for the Acting Administrator of the Agency for International Development

Subject: AID Family Planning Grants/Mexico City Policy

The Foreign Assistance Act of 1961 prohibits nongovernmental organizations ("NGO's") that receive Federal funds from using those funds "to pay for the performance of abortions as a method of family planning, or to motivate or coerce any person to practice abortions." (22 U.S.C. 215lb(f)(1)). The August 1984 announcement by President Reagan of what has become know as the "Mexico City Policy" directed the Agency for International Development ("AID") to expand this limitation and withhold AID funds from NGO's that engage in a wide range of activities, including providing advice, counseling, or information regarding abortion, or lobbying a foreign government to legalize or make abortion available. These conditions have been imposed even where an NGO uses non-AID funds for abortion-related activities.

These excessively broad anti-abortion conditions are unwarranted. I am informed that the conditions are not mandated by the Foreign Assistance Act or any other law. Moreover, they have undermined efforts to promote safe and efficacious family planning programs in foreign nations. Accordingly, I hereby direct that AID remove the conditions not explicitly mandated by the Foreign Assistance Act or any other law from all current AID grants to NGO's and exclude them from future grants.

PRESIDENT GEORGE W. BUSH'S POLICY

Memorandum for the Administrator of the United States Agency for International Development.
"The President: Memorandum of March 28, 2001; Restoration of the Mexico City Policy," Federal Register, Vol. 66, No. 61 (March 29, 2001), 17303–13.

Subject: Restoration of the Mexico City Policy

The Mexico City Policy announced by President Reagan in 1984 required nongovernmental organizations to agree as a condition of their receipt of Federal funds that such organizations would neither perform nor actively promote abortion as a method of family planning in other nations. This policy was in effect until it was rescinded on January 22, 1993.

It is my conviction that taxpayer funds should not be used to pay for abortions or advocate or actively promote abortion, either here or abroad. It is therefore my belief that the Mexico City Policy should be restored. Accordingly, I hereby rescind the "Memorandum for the Acting Administrator for the Agency for International Development, Subject: AID Family Planning Grants/Mexico City Policy," dated January 22, 1993, and I direct the Administrator of the United States Agency for International Development to reinstate in full all of the requirements of the Mexico City Policy in effect on January 19, 1993.

PRESIDENT BARACK OBAMA'S POLICY

Mexico City Policy—Voluntary Population Planning
Memorandum for the Secretary of State, the Administrator of the United States Agency for International Development

"Presidential Documents: Memorandum of January 23, 2009; Memorandum on Mexico City Policy and Assistance for Voluntary Population Planning," *Federal Register* 74, no. 17 (January 28, 2009): 4903–4.

Subject: Mexico City Policy and Assistance for Voluntary Population Planning
THE WHITE HOUSE, January 23, 2009.

The Foreign Assistance Act of 1961 (22 U.S.C. 2151b(f)(1)), prohibits non-governmental organizations (NGOs) that receive Federal funds from using those funds "to pay for the performance of abortions as a method of family planning, or to motivate or coerce any person to practice abortions." The August 1984 announcement by President Reagan of what has become known as the "Mexico City Policy" directed the United States Agency for International Development (USAID) to expand this limitation and withhold USAID funds from NGOs that use non-USAID funds to engage in a wide range of activities, including providing advice, counseling, or information regarding abortion, or lobbying a foreign government to legalize or make abortion available. The Mexico City Policy was in effect from 1985 until 1993, when it was rescinded by President Clinton. President George W. Bush reinstated the policy in 2001, implementing it through conditions in USAID grant awards, and subsequently extended the policy to "voluntary population planning" assistance provided by the Department of State.

These excessively broad conditions on grants and assistance awards are unwarranted. Moreover, they have undermined efforts to promote safe and effective voluntary family planning programs in foreign nations. Accordingly, I hereby revoke the Presidential memorandum of January 22, 2001, for the Administrator of USAID (Restoration of the Mexico City Policy), the Presidential memorandum of March 28, 2001, for the Administrator of USAID (Restoration of the Mexico City Policy), and the Presidential memorandum of August 29, 2003, for the Secretary of State (Assistance for Voluntary Population Planning). In addition, I direct the Secretary of State and the Administrator of USAID to take the following actions with respect to conditions in voluntary population planning assistance and USAID grants that were imposed pursuant to either the 2001 or 2003 memoranda and that are not required by the Foreign Assistance Act or any other law: (1) immediately waive such conditions in any current grants, and (2) notify current grantees, as soon as possible, that these conditions have been waived. I further direct that the Department of State and USAID immediately cease imposing these conditions in any future grants.

This memorandum is not intended to, and does not, create any right or benefit, substantive or procedural, enforceable at law or in equity by any party against the United States, its departments, agencies, or entities, its officers, employees, or agents, or any other person.

The Secretary of State is authorized and directed to publish this memorandum in the *Federal Register.*

Timeline for Birth Control Issues

Sixteenth century	Condoms made of animal membrane are first introduced in Paris.
1798	Thomas Malthus publishes *An Essay on the Principles of Population*, which sets forth the principle that unrestrained population can be harmful to society. This concept later becomes the fundamental premise behind a multitude of family planning ideologies.
1823	Francis Place hands out flyers in England describing the use of sea sponges as an inexpensive pessary.
1826	Richard Carlile publishes the first English-language pamphlet on contraceptives titled *What Is Love?*
1832	Charles Knowlton is convicted three times for publishing a birth control manual in the Massachusetts, *The Fruits of Philosophy*.
1843	Charles Goodyear invents the vulcanization process to make rubber more flexible to use with cervical caps, diaphragms, and rubber condoms
1873	Congress passes the Comstock Law, making it a felony to sell, publish, or otherwise distribute pornography, including contraceptive manuals.
1881	Ohio doctor S. S. Lungren performs the first tubal ligation.

1883	The Woman's Christian Temperance Union forms the Department for the Promotion of Purity in Literature and Art.
1883	The cousin of Charles Darwin, Francis Galton, publishes *Inquiries into Human Faculty and Its Development* introducing the scientific theory of eugenics.
1897	H. D. Lennander performs the first vasectomy on humans in Sweden.
1899	Harry Sharp of Indiana State Reformatory begins performing vasectomies on inmates.
1907	Indiana legislature passes law authorizing involuntary sterilization of certain classes of criminals, feebleminded dependents, and habitual criminals. Over the next 20 years, nearly half of all states follow Indiana's example.
1909	Richard Richter invents first intrauterine device (IUD).
1914	Margaret Sanger coins the term "birth control" in her magazine *The Woman Rebel—No Gods, No Masters.*
1915	Mary Ware Dennett forms the National Birth Control League, which later becomes the Voluntary Parenthood League.
1921	Margaret Sanger forms the American Birth Control League dedicated to promoting the legalization and dissemination of birth control information and devices.
1921	Margaret Sanger initiates a debate in the *New York Times* editorial page with Catholic Archbishop Patrick Hayes, that eventually results in a shift in Protestant views of birth control.
1925	Robert Latou Dickinson forms the Committee on Maternal Health.
1926	American Eugenics Society forms in the United States to organize legal policies to ensure "responsible" reproduction.
1927	U.S. Supreme Court affirms the constitutionality of involuntary sterilization for certain classes of inmates in *Buck v. Bell* decision.
1928	Ernst Grafenberg markets a modified IUD using a silk wrapped silver ring.
1928	Margaret Sanger forms the Clinical Research Bureau and the Committee of Federal Legislation.
1930	The Northern Baptist Conference becomes the first mainline protestant denomination to formally tolerate the use of birth control in the United States.

1930	The Anglican Church Conference in Lambeth, England, passes a resolution explicitly permitting the use of contraceptives affecting Protestants worldwide.
1930	Pope Pius XI promulgates an encyclical on Christian marriage, *Casti Connubii*, which reaffirms the Catholic view that artificial contraception is a "sin against God."
1936	A federal circuit court rules in *U.S. v. One Package of Japanese Pessaries* that doctors can prescribe contraceptives in their offices without violating Comstock's prohibiting of obscenity.
1942	The Supreme Court rules in *Skinner v. Oklahoma* that sterilization may not be imposed as a criminal penalty.
1942	Three separate birth control organizations founded by Margaret Sanger, Mary Ware Dennett, and Robert Dickinson combine resources to form Planned Parenthood Federation of America.
1957	Gregory Pincus, John Rock, and Christopher Tietze discover an anovulent oral contraceptive and begin testing a commercial version.
1958	Lazar Marguilies introduces a spiral or coil-shaped IUD.
1958	Sweden becomes the first Western nation to contribute funds toward family planning programs in a colonial state as part of its foreign policy objectives.
1960	The Food and Drug Administration (FDA) approves the first progestin/estrogen combination oral contraceptive, which is more commonly known as "the pill."
1961	The General Board of the National Council of Churches of Christ issues a statement permitting couples freedom to use contraceptives as a medical treatment.
1965	The Supreme Court rules in *Griswold v. Connecticut* that married persons have a constitutional "right to privacy," including decisions regarding regulation of birth. The ruling strikes down existing state statutes outlawing sale and distribution of contraceptives.
1967	President Lyndon Johnson signs the Social Security Amendments of 1967, which stipulates that at least 6 percent of maternal and child health care funds be spent on family planning services.
1968	Howard Tatum introduces a T-shaped IUD.
1968	Pope Paul VI promulgates *Humanae Vitae*, which explicitly reaffirms the Catholic Church's view that both artificial contraceptives and induced abortions are grave sins.

1968   Canadian Conference of Catholic Bishops releases the
                "Winnipeg Statement," which asserts that individual
                Catholics can choose to accept *Humanae Vitae* according
                to their individual conscience. This creates the basis for a
                rift within the Catholic Church over the issue of artificial
                birth control.

1970   President Richard Nixon signs Title X of the Public
                Health Service Act, creating the first federal program
                devoted entirely to birth control services.

1971   A. H. Robins Company introduces the Dalkon Shield.

1973   The FDA approves a progestin-only hormone "minipill."

1973   The Supreme Court expands the "right to privacy" doc-
                trine, initially formed by *Griswold*, to include a woman's
                right to procure an abortion.

1974   The FDA suspends support for the Dalkon Shield brand of
                IUD after receiving reports of spontaneous abortions and
                deaths related to the product.

1977   The first "Hyde Amendment" is adopted by Congress to
                prohibit federal dollars for family planning from being
                used for abortion services.

1979   China institutes a "one-child" policy mandating universal
                birth control in an effort to reduce the possibility of
                overpopulation.

1980   Etienne-Emile Baulieu develops a steroid that blocks the
                effects of progesterone, which effectively ends embryo
                development in the uterus. The abortifacient is code-
                named RU-486 and later marketed under the name of
                Mifepristone. It is used to induce nonsurgical abortion.

1981   President Ronald Reagan signs the Adolescent Family
                Life Act, which provides federal funding for family plan-
                ning programs that discourage premarital sexuality and
                that promote adoption instead of abortion.

1984   President Ronald Reagan announces the "Mexico City
                Policy," which prohibits federal family planning funds
                from being used for abortion services.

1987   The first legal condom commercial airs on television in
                San Francisco.

1990   The FDA approves the first long-acting contraceptive
                facilitated through a subdermal implant. It is marketed
                under the brand name Norplant.

1992	The FDA approves the first injectable long-term contraceptive, which is marketed under the brand name Depo-Provera.
1993	President Bill Clinton reverses the Mexico City Policy enacted during the Reagan and Bush administrations.
1999	The FDA approves the first "emergency contraceptive," which is marketed under the brand Plan B.
2001	President George W. Bush reinstates the Mexico City Policy that had been rescinded during the Clinton administration.
2002	The FDA approves a minimally invasive surgical implant called the Essure System, which renders permanent sterilization in women.
2002	President George W. Bush launches a well-funded federal program promoting "abstinence only" as a primary means of birth control.
2003	The FDA approves a low-dose daily oral contraceptive that reduces the frequency of menstruation to once every three months. It is marketed under the name Seasonale.
2006	The FDA approves the sales of Plan B for women over the age of 18, without a prescription.
2007	The FDA approves a low-dose oral contraceptive marketed under the brand name Lybrel, which eliminates all menstruation cycles.
2009	President Barack Obama reverses the Mexico City Policy of the Bush administration.
2009	Congress passes a federal conscience clause provision, which extends to doctors, pharmacies, and other health entities the right to refuse to provide contraceptive services for moral and religious reasons.

GLOSSARY

Abortifacient: Any mechanical or chemical means that induces an embryonic abortion after the sperm successfully passes into the uterus and fertilizes the ovum. It is often caused by a failure of the ovum to attach itself to the walls of the uterus.

Abortion: The premature destruction of the fertilized ovum regardless of cause. More commonly, the term refers to any deliberate termination of a pregnancy (an induced abortion). A spontaneous, or accidental, abortion is usually identified as a miscarriage.

Age of Consent: A legal term that refers to the age at which the state deems a child is mature enough to make an informed decision without the consent of their legal guardians. Ages may differ depending on the type of decision. The age at which a state allows a girl to make decisions about medical options (including contraceptives) may not be the same age at which it allows them to consent to sexual intercourse.

Antiandrogenic: A drug that blocks the production of male sex hormones. It is an active feature in the Yaz/Yasmin brand of contraceptives used to prevent acne.

Antimineralocorticoid: A drug that counteracts water and sodium retention. It is an active feature in the Yaz/Yasmin brand of contraceptives used to prevent bloating and other aches related to premenstrual dysphoric disorder.

Artificial Birth Control: Any mechanical or chemical means used to prevent the conception of an ovum during or after intercourse. These methods rely not on the timing of sexual intercourse but on the barrier or chemical prevention.

Bilateral Salpingo-Oophorectomy: The surgical removal of ovaries and both fallopian tubes that results in complete sterilization in women.

Birth Control: Any deliberate attempt to prevent conception. The term may be used to refer to both artificial and natural methods of contraception, though it most often refers to artificial methods.

Castration: Any action, surgical or chemical, that eliminates the functions of the testicles, resulting in complete sterilization for men.

Combination Pill: The first form of oral contraceptive introduced in 1960 that combines progestin and estrogen hormones to prevent ovulation. The drug ensures that the ovum is never released to the ovaries so that pregnancy cannot occur. It is popularly known as "the pill."

Comstock Law: A federal law passed in 1873 that prohibited the transmission of indecent materials through the postal system. The definition of "indecent" was sufficiently broad to include the transmission of materials related to contraception. Most states passed similar "Comstock laws."

Condom: A method of contraception relying on a physical barrier to prevent direct contact between the semen and the vagina. Male condoms are most common, comprised of an impermeable sheath that fits over the penis. Female condoms are less common, utilizing larger a sheath that fits into the vagina prior to sexual contact.

Conscience Clause: Legal protection for doctors or other medical entities who choose not to dispense advice or treatments that are contrary to their religious or philosophical beliefs. Prevents legal liability for doctors who refuse to perform abortions or prescribe/provide contraceptives.

Contraceptive: Any method used to prevent the fertilization of the ovum during or after sexual intercourse. Common referred to as "birth control," which is subdivided into natural and artificial methods.

Dalkon Shield: The brand name of an intrauterine device introduced by the A. H. Robins Company in 1971. The Food and Drug Administration suspended support in 1974 because of the high number of side effects, which included spontaneous abortions and death.

Depo-Provera: The brand name of a long-acting contraception based on a synthetic progesterone hormone called medroxyprogesterone introduced in 1997. The product was the first injectable contraceptive providing contraception for three months.

Diaphragm: A rubber device inserted inside the vagina that is used to create a barrier between sperm and the uterus during sexual contact. Referred to as a pessary prior to the twentieth century. Similar in function to cervical caps, sponges, and other contraceptive barrier devices.

Drospirenone: A synthetic form of progestogen used in combination with ethanol estradiol as a contraceptive. The active ingredient in the Yaz/Yasmin brand of contraceptives because it contains antiandrogenic and antimineralocorticoid properties.

Emergency Contraceptive: Commonly used to describe any contraceptive designed to be used after sexual contact. It is not clear if existing postcoital products act as contraceptives or abortifacients.

Essure System: A method of sterilization for women that involves a small metal implant inserted into the fallopian tubes by means of a catheter. It is considered minor surgery.

Eugenics: A spectrum of scientific theories developed in the late 1800s that believed that a more perfect human race could be crafted from careful manipulation of human breeding.

Guaranteed Access to Prescription: A legislative action that holds doctors and other medical entities liable to civil rights–based litigation if they refuse to carry or dispense contraceptives. Passed by several states but never passed at the federal level.

Hormonal-Based Contraceptives: A form of artificial contraception that relies on chemical interactions to interrupt either the ovulation or the fertilization process in order to prevent pregnancy. Interruption of the implantation process after fertilization changes a contraceptive to an abortifacient.

Intrauterine Device: A coil, loop, triangle, or T-shaped device made out of plastic or metal that is inserted into the uterus to prevent conception. Scientists are unsure whether the material or the shape is responsible for the contraception, which may last for many years.

Lactational Amenorrhea Method: A method of natural contraception that involves extending the duration of breast feeding to postpone ovulation. This method is typically used to ensure minimal "spacing" between the births.

Lambeth Decision: A resolution passed in 1930 by the international Anglican Church Conference in Lambeth, England, that formally tolerated the use of contraceptives among church members.

Levonorgestrel: A synthetic form for progestin that can be dispensed in low doses over a very long period of time. The active ingredient in the Norplant System.

Long-Acting Hormone-Based Contraceptives: A form of artificial contraceptive that is given to the patient once but then dispenses low doses of steroidal hormones over a long period of time. Effective durations depend on the delivery system: patches may last one week, injections might last one month, while some implants can last for as long as five years.

Lunelle: The brand name of an injectable form of long-acting hormonal contraceptive that was introduced in 2000. The synthetic progestrin and estrogen combination lasts for one month.

Lybrel: The brand name of a low-dose oral hormone-based contraceptive that may be taken 365 days a year without the need for placebo pills. Introduced in 2007, the product eliminates monthly menstruation cycles.

Mifepristone: The brand name for a steroid that blocks the development of progesterone, which is necessary for a fertilized ovum to survive. The drug was developed in France under the code name RU-486 and was approved in the United States in 1996 for the purpose of inducing nonsurgical abortions.

Minilaparotomy: A less intrusive form of surgical operation to bind fallopian tubes together for female sterilization. The process is performed through very small slits in the abdomen.

Minipill: A form of oral contraceptive that relies on a progestin-only hormone to reduce and thicken the cervical mucus to prevent sperm from reaching the uterus. Unlike the combination pill, the minipill does not affect the ovulation process.

Natural Birth Control Methods: Natural methods of contraception do not involve any outside chemical or device to implement and rely exclusively on the restraint of the individual sexual partners to abstain or limit sexual activity during times when conception is most likely.

Natural Family Planning: The only method of natural birth control permitted by the Catholic Church. It involves restricting the timing of sexual activity only to those days of postovulation. Several methods may be used for determining the days of ovulation, including daily monitoring of cervical mucus or the sympto-thermal monitoring system.

Nongovernmental Organizations: Any private organization composed of legal citizens outside the explicit auspices of any single government. Such organizations are often funded by governments to promote policies without having to bear the responsibility of direct implementation. International family planning programs are most often carried out through these organizations.

Norplant System: The brand name of a long-acting hormone-based contraceptive that was introduced in 1990. The device consisted of six rods implanted just below the skin that released low doses of levonorgestrel to sustain contraception for up to five years. Manufacturers pulled the product from the market in 2002 after numerous reports of harsh side effects.

NuvaRing: The brand name of a plastic ring-shaped intrauterine device introduced in 2001. The product also releases low doses of progestin and estrogen for three weeks at a time. It must be removed prior to menstruation.

Ortho Evra: The brand name of a low-dose hormone-based long-acting contraceptive delivered through a patch that is affixed to the skin. Introduced in 2001, the patch is effective for a week at a time.

Pessaries: An archaic term used to describe a rubber barrier inserted into the vagina to prevent sperm from reaching the uterus. The modern term for such a device is diaphragm. Current usage refers to a plastic ring set inside the vagina to treat certain disorders related to prolapsed uterus and may or may not include contraceptive properties.

The Pill: The popular name for the first oral contraceptive, which was a combination pill approved by the Food and Drug Administration in 1960.

Premenstrual Dysphoric Disorder: A combination of symptoms that occur just prior to a woman's monthly menstruation cycle. Indications associated with increased water retention prior to ovulation include backaches, stomach cramps, headaches, tenderness in the breasts, and increased nervousness and irritability.

Preven (Plan B): The brand name for the first contraceptive intended to be effective after sexual contact. Introduced in 1999, the drug suppresses the mid-cycle leuteinizing hormone surge that triggers ovulation. Scientists cannot confirm whether the drug is a true contraceptive or whether it is an abortifacient that acts after fertilization.

Pro-Choice: A term used to describe a broad spectrum of ideologies that promotes complete individual autonomy over questions of reproduction. Most commonly refers to specific support for a woman's right to induce abortion but may also refer to a sociopolitical movement that supports less restrictive definitions of parenthood, family, and sexuality.

Pro-Family: A term used to describe a broad spectrum of ideologies that promotes monogamous heterosexual family structures as the primary unit in society. Commonly refers to a sociopolitical movement that supports parental rights and opposes abortion, same-sex marriage, extramarital sexual relations, and no-fault divorce. Birth control may or may not be supported.

Progressive Era: A term commonly used to describe a period in American history between 1895 and 1915. Progressive ideologies included a broad spectrum of priorities but generally promoted the use of scientific methodologies to solve social problems through local government.

Race Suicide: An archaic term used by eugenicists around the turn of the twentieth century to describe the consequence of unrestricted reproduction among certain groups overwhelming the low birthrates among established families. It was based on a fear that the unimpeded growth of lesser quality populations would undermine the quality of human stock. It is not necessarily related to ethnicity, but it did refer to threats from lower social classes.

Republican Motherhood: An ideological concept among Americans around the turn of the nineteenth century that emphasized the critical role of mothers in educating children to be intelligent citizens in a democratic society. Motherhood was promoted as an active vocation necessary to protecting free society from devolving into a self-serving tyranny of the majority.

Seasonale: The brand name of a low-dose daily combination pill introduced in 2003. The oral contraceptive was the first brand to be marketed for its ability to limit menstruation cycles to once every three months.

Sterilization: Any action that renders a man or woman permanently incapable of conception. Sterilization may be accidental or deliberate. The most common method for deliberate sterilization in men is a surgical vasectomy, and the most common method for women is surgical tubal ligation. Other nonsurgical methods exist through chemical or mechanical means.

Sympto-Thermal Method: A system used within the natural family planning method of birth control that combines daily monitoring of cervical mucus with daily readings of basal body temperatures to determine days of ovulation.

Temperance: An ideological concept among Americans that emphasized the value of individual moral restraint. It was prominent during the last half of the nineteenth century and was commonly used to describe the opposition to excessive consumption of alcohol. It was also the basis for social policies targeting a wide variety of moral vices, including the prohibition of the dissemination of contraceptive literature and devices.

Tubal Ligation: A method of surgical sterilization used for women to permanently prevent conception. The fallopian tubes, which connect the ovaries to the uterus, are bound together in two places, and the sections in between are removed.

Vasectomy: A method of surgical sterilization used for men to permanently prevent conception. The small duct that carries sperm from the testes to the urethra is cut, cauterized, or otherwise obstructed.

Voluntariness: A concept that refers to an individual's willingness to participate in an activity, involving a free-will decision without outside pressure or coercion.

Yasmin: The brand name of a drospirenone-based contraceptive introduced to the market by Berlex Laboratories in 2003. The drug was unique for receiving Food and Drug Administration approval for multiple uses in addition to its contraceptive properties, including treatment for premenstrual dysmorphic disorder and for treating acne. Yasmin was formulated for a 28-day cycle.

Yaz: The brand name of a drospirenone-based contraceptive introduced to the market by Berlex Laboratories in 2003. The drug was unique for receiving Food and Drug Administration approval for multiple uses in addition to its contraceptive properties, including treatment for premenstrual dysmorphic disorder and for treating acne. Yaz was formulated for a 24-day cycle.

FURTHER READING

Ashton, James. *The Book of Nature: Containing Information for Young People Who Think of Getting Married, on the Philosophy of Procreation and Sexual Intercourse; Showing How to Prevent Conception and to Avoid Child-Bearing; Also, Rules for Management During Labor and Child-Birth*. New York, 1865.

Bennett, Jane, and Alexandra Pope. *The Pill: Are You Sure It's for You?* St. Leonards: Allen & Unwin, 2009.

Bernards, Neal, and Lynn Hall, eds. *Teenage Sexuality: Opposing Viewpoints*. San Diego: Greenhaven Press, 1988.

Capo, Beth Widmaier. *Textual Contraception: Birth Control and Modern American Fiction*, Columbus: Ohio State University Press, 2007.

Caron, Simone M. *Who Chooses? American Reproductive History since 1830*. Gainesville: University Press of Florida, 2008.

Cassidy, Keith. "The Right to Life Movement: Sources, Development, and Strategies." In *The Politics of Abortion and Birth Control in Historical Perspective*, edited by Donald Critchlow. University Park: Pennsylvania State University Press, 1996, 128–59.

Critchlow, Donald. "Birth Control, Population Control, and Family Planning: An Overview." In *The Politics of Abortion and Birth Control in Historical Perspective*. University Park: Pennsylvania State University Press, 1996, 1–21.

Dennett, Mary Ware. *Birth Control Laws: Shall We Keep Them, Change Them, or Abolish Them?* New York: Da Capo Press, 1970.

Devettere, Raymond J. *Practical Decision Making in Health Care Ethics: Cases and Concepts*. Washington, DC: Georgetown University Press, 2010.

Dienes, C. Thomas. *Law, Politics and Birth Control.* Chicago: University of Illinois Press, 1972.

Dowbiggin, Ian. *The Sterilization Movement and Global Fertility in the Twentieth Century.* New York: Oxford University Press, 2008.

Dudley, William, ed. *Reproductive Rights.* Farmington Hills, MI: Greenhaven Press, 2006.

Fielding, Michael, *Parenthood: Design or Accident—A Manual of Birth Control.* New York: Vanguard Press, 1935.

Foote, Edward B. *The Radical Remedy in Social Science: Or, Borning Better Babies through Regulating Reproduction by Controlling Conception; An Earnest Essay on Pressing Problems.* New York, 1889.

Foote, Edward B. *Reproductive Control: Or, a Rational Guide to Matrimonial Happiness; The Right and Duty of Parents to Limit the Number of Their Offspring According to Their Circumstances Demonstrated; A Brief Account of All Known Modes of Preventing Conception with Their Physical and Social Effects; By An American Physician.* Cincinnati, 1855.

Franks, Angela. *Margaret Sanger's Eugenic Legacy: The Control of Female Fertility.* Jefferson, NC: McFarland, 2005.

Gerber-Fried, Marlene. *From Abortion to Reproductive Freedom: Transforming a Movement.* Boston: South End Press, 1990.

Gordon, Linda. *The Moral Property of Women: A History of Birth Control Politics in America.* Chicago: University of Illinois Press, 2002.

Gordon, Linda. *Woman's Body, Woman's Right: Birth Control in America.* New York: Penguin Books, 1990.

Guillebaud, John. *The Pill and Other Hormonal Contraceptives.* New York: Oxford University Press, 2005.

Guttmacher, Alan F. *The Complete Book of Birth Control.* New York: Ballantine Books, 1968.

Hull, N. E. H., William James Hoffer, and Peter Charles Hoffer. *The Abortion Rights Controversy in America: A Legal Reader.* Chapel Hill: University of North Carolina Press, 2004.

Hunter, James Davison, and Joseph E. Davis. "Cultural Politics at the Edge of Life." In *The Politics of Abortion and Birth Control in Historical Perspective*, edited by Donald Critchlow. University Park: Pennsylvania State University Press, 1996, 103–27.

Johnson, John W. *Griswold v. Connecticut: Birth Control and the Constitutional Right of Privacy.* Lawrence University Press of Kansas, 2005.

Kasun, Jacqueline *The War against Population: The Economics and Ideology of World Population Control.* San Francisco: Ignatius Press, 1999.

Kevles, Daniel J. *In the Name of Eugenics: Genetics and the Uses of Human Heredity,* Berkeley: University of California Press, 1985.

Kluchin, Rebecca M. *Fit to Be Tied: Sterilization and Reproductive Rights in America, 1950–1980.* New Brunswick, NJ: Rutgers University Press, 2009.

Mastroianni, Luigi, Peter J. Donaldson, and Thomas T. Kane. *Developing New Contraceptives: Obstacles and Opportunities* Washington, DC: National Academy Press, 1990.

Monsma, John Clover. *Religion and Birth Control: Twenty-One Medical Specialists Write in Plain Language about Control of Conception, Therapeutic Abortion, Sterilization, Natural Childbirth, Artificial Insemination.* Garden City, NY: Doubleday, 1963.

Montgomery, John Warwick. *Slaughter of the Innocents: Abortion, Birth Control, and Divorce in Light of Science, Law and Theology.* Westchester, IL: Crossway Books, 1981.

Mosher, Steven W. *Population Control: Real Costs—Illusory Benefits.* New Brunswick, NJ: Transaction, 2008.

Moskowitz, Ellen H., and Bruce Jennings. *Coerced Contraception? Moral and Policy Challenges of Long-Acting Birth Control.* Washington, DC: Georgetown University Press, 1996.

Mylchreest, Ian. "'Sound Law and Undoubtedly Good Policy': *Roe v. Wade* in Comparative Perspective." In *The Politics of Abortion and Birth Control in Historical Perspective*, edited by Donald Critchlow. University Park: Pennsylvania State University Press, 1996, 53–71.

Nelson, Jennifer. *Women of Color and the Reproductive Rights Movement.* New York: New York University Press, 2003.

Perkins, Barbara Bridgman, *Adolescent Birth Planning and Sexuality: Abstracts of the Literature.* Washington, DC: Consortium on Early Childbearing and Childrearing Child Welfare League of America, 1974.

Reed, James W. "The Birth-Control Movement before *Roe v. Wade.*" In *The Politics of Abortion and Birth Control in Historical Perspective*, edited by Donald Critchlow. University Park: Pennsylvania State University Press, 1996, 22–52.

Reed, James W. *From Private Vice to Public Virtue: The Birth Control Movement and American Society since 1830.* New York: Basic Books, 1978.

Roberts, Dorothy. *Killing the Black Body: Race, Reproduction, and the Meaning of Liberty.* New York: Vintage Books, 1997.

Rock, John, *The Time Has Come: A Catholic Doctor's Proposals to End the Battle over Birth Control.* New York: Alfred A. Knopf, 1963.

Rosen, Christine. *Preaching Eugenics: Religious Leaders and the American Eugenics Movement.* New York: Oxford University Press, 2004.

Rosenberg, Charles, and Carroll Smith-Rosenberg, eds. *Birth Control and Family Planning in Nineteenth Century America.* New York: Arno Press, 1974.

Rowland, Debran. *Boundaries of Her Body: The Troubling History of Women's Rights in America.* Naperville, IL: Sphinx, 2004.

Sharpless, John. "World Population Growth, Family Planning, and American Foreign Policy." In *The Politics of Abortion and Birth Control in Historical Perspective*, edited by Donald Critchlow. University Park: Pennsylvania State University Press, 1996, 72–102.

Soule, J. *Science of Reproduction and Reproductive Control: The Necessity of Some Abstaining from Having Children.* New York, 1856.

Staggenborg, Suzanne. "The Survival of the Pro-Choice Movement." In *The Politics of Abortion and Birth Control in Historical Perspective*, edited by Donald Critchlow. University Park: Pennsylvania State University Press, 1996, 160–76.

Strasburger, Victor C., Barbara J. Wilson, and Amy Beth Jordan. *Children, Adolescents, and the Media.* 2nd ed. Thousand Oaks, CA: Sage, 2009.

Tentler, Leslie Woodcock. *Catholics and Contraception: An American History.* Ithaca, NY: Cornell University Press, 2004.

Throne, Barrie, and Marilyn Yalom, eds. *Rethinking the Family: Some Feminist Questions.* Boston: Northeastern University Press, 1992.

Tobin, Kathleen A. *The American Religious Debate over Birth Control, 1907–1937.* Jefferson, NC: McFarland, 2001.

Tone, Andrea. *Devices and Desires: A History of Contraceptives in America.* New York: Hill and Wang, 2001.

Tone, Andrea, ed. *Controlling Reproduction: An American History.* Wilmington, DE: Scholarly Resources Inc., 1997.

Walsh-Childers, Kim, Alyse Gotthoffer, Debbie Treise, and Carolyn Ringer. "From 'Just the Facts' to 'Downright Salacious': Teen and Women's Magazines' Coverage of Sex and Sexual Health." In *Sexual Teens, Sexual Media*, edited by Jane Brown, Jeanne Steele, and Kim Walsh-Childers. Mahwah, NJ: Lawrence Erlbaum Associates, 2002.

Weisbord, Robert G. *Genocide? Birth Control and the Black American.* Westport, CT: Greenwood Press, 1975.

Wekesser, Carol, ed. *Feminism: Opposing Viewpoints.* San Diego: Greenhaven Press, 1995.

INDEX

About the Author

Aharon W. Zorea is associate professor in history at the University of Wisconsin, Richland, WI. His specialties include 20th-century American politics, law, and social policy. His published works include *In the Image of God: A Christian Response to Capital Punishment.*